RANJIT KUMAR

Diabetes Habits

Transforming Your Health One Tiny Habit at a Time

First edition

This book was professionally typeset on Reedsy.
Find out more at reedsy.com

Contents

Introduction

Whenever someone checks their blood sugar, they often remember the first time it spiked—hearts racing as they stare at the numbers, feeling a wave of helplessness. That moment sparked their journey towards understanding that small changes can lead to big health transformations. This book is born from countless stories like these, where individuals just like you faced moments of uncertainty and decided to take control of their health. You're not alone on this path; whether you've been managing diabetes for years or are just starting to encounter its challenges, we understand what you're going through.

Diabetes management can feel overwhelming. The sheer volume of information, dietary restrictions, exercise recommendations, and medication schedules can be daunting. Yet, the good news is that it's the small, manageable tweaks in our everyday habits that hold remarkable power. A sip of water before a meal, a few minutes of gentle stretching, or opting to walk a block longer than usual—these might seem insignificant, but they accumulate into meaningful progress over time. When I delved into the world of health and wellness, I discovered the transformative power of tiny habits. Just like a single drop of water can create ripples, a single, mindful choice can set into motion a cascade of positive health changes.

The beauty of these micro-habits lies in their simplicity. They don't require drastic lifestyle overhauls or heroic willpower. Instead, they are small shifts in daily life that, when practiced consistently, result in profound health benefits. For those managing diabetes, these shifts can mean the difference between feeling overwhelmed and feeling empowered. Imagine making small, strategic changes seamlessly integrated into your regular routine. These are easy to remember, simple to practice, and incredibly effective. Before long, you'll notice improvements that not only make diabetes management easier but also enhance your overall quality of life.

Consider the concept of micro-habits like planting seeds. Each small change acts as a seed that, when nurtured, grows into a robust plant. Imagine taking just a few minutes daily to focus on a healthier lifestyle. Those minutes add up, translating into hours, weeks, and months of mindful living. Over time, these small efforts collectively bring about significant improvements in managing your diabetes.

Throughout this book, you'll find actionable steps and real-life examples that show how simple changes—like swapping one sugary snack for a healthier option—can lead to improved blood sugar control and overall wellness. We're here to guide you through every step, providing practical advice, motivational stories, and evidence-based strategies tailored to your specific needs. You'll learn about the importance of nutrition, the role of physical activity, the impact of stress management, and how to maintain a positive mindset.

Our journey together will start with the basics: understanding diabetes. We'll discuss what happens inside your body when you have diabetes, explaining it in clear, easy-to-understand terms. Then, we'll move on to the significance of diet and how choosing the right foods can make a substantial difference in controlling your blood sugar levels. You don't need to give up everything you love—it's about finding a balance that works for you.

Exercise doesn't mean exhausting workouts. Even light activities like gardening, dancing, or walking can greatly benefit your health. We've included exercises that can easily fit into your daily schedule, keeping in mind any mobility issues or other health concerns you might have. Stress can significantly impact diabetes, and learning to manage it is crucial. This book will provide techniques to help you relax and reduce anxiety, contributing to better health management.

Moreover, we'll explore the emotional aspects of living with diabetes. It's normal to feel frustrated, anxious, or even depressed sometimes. Acknowledging these feelings and finding ways to cope can empower you to face diabetes with a stronger, more positive outlook. We'll also offer support for caregivers and family members, recognizing their critical role in helping loved ones manage their condition effectively.

You'll learn about the latest research and innovations in diabetes care, presented in an accessible manner. We'll demystify new treatments and technologies, giving you the information needed to make informed decisions about your health. Whether it's continuous glucose monitors, insulin pumps, or emerging medications, you'll be equipped with knowledge to discuss options with your healthcare provider confidently.

As part of this holistic approach, we've included checklists, planning tools, and templates to help you implement the advised changes smoothly. Keeping track of your progress will become second nature, and you'll continually see how these small adjustments impact your health positively. Every chapter concludes with a summary and key takeaways to reinforce what you've learned and keep you focused on your goals.

This book aims to build a community of individuals supporting each other, sharing experiences, and encouraging one another. By reading the personal stories of people who have successfully managed their diabetes through micro-habits, you'll find inspiration and realize that you too can achieve similar results.

Finally, we'll delve into how healthcare professionals can support you on this journey. Effective communication with your doctor, discussing concerns openly, and working collaboratively are vital elements in managing diabetes successfully. You'll gain insights into how to advocate for yourself, ensuring you receive the best possible care tailored to your unique needs.

In conclusion, this book provides you with the knowledge and tools needed to navigate your diabetes management journey confidently. With each page, you'll discover that small, consistent actions lead to significant health improvements over time. Let's embark on this journey together, embracing the power of micro-habits to transform your health and well-being.

1

Understanding the Power of Tiny Habits

Understanding the power of tiny habits can make a significant difference in managing diabetes, especially for seniors. This chapter delves into how small, manageable changes in daily routines can lead to substantial health improvements over time. By focusing on micro-habits, such as drinking more water or taking short walks, individuals can incorporate healthy behaviors without feeling overwhelmed. These small steps create a foundation for lasting change, promoting better glucose control and overall well-being. Through regular practice of these tiny habits, one can build resilience and establish a routine that makes healthy living second nature.

In this chapter, you will discover how behavioral psychology underpins the formation of tiny habits, emphasizing the roles of triggers and rewards in embedding new behaviors. We will also explore the physiological impact of minor lifestyle adjustments on diabetes management, supported by scientific research and real-life success stories. You'll learn about the brain's ability to adapt through neuroplasticity, making repeated actions automatic over time. Additionally, practical applications tailored to individual motivators will be discussed, including the importance of creating a supportive environment and involving family members in the journey towards healthier living. The goal is to provide you with actionable strategies that are easy to implement, helping you or your loved ones manage diabetes more effectively through consistent, small changes.

The Science Behind Tiny Habits

Understanding how tiny habits can aid in diabetes management involves delving into both psychological and physiological foundations. This section explains how small, manageable changes can bring about significant improvements in health, particularly for seniors managing diabetes.

Tiny habits form through principles grounded in behavioral psychology. Essentially, when a small action is performed repeatedly under the right conditions, it becomes a lasting habit. Triggers and rewards play crucial roles here. A trigger could be something as simple as placing a glass of water beside your bed to prompt drinking water first thing in the morning. The reward might be the refreshing feeling after hydrating, encouraging you to repeat the action daily. Over time, these consistent repetitions embed the behavior, making it an automatic part of your routine.

Health impact research supports the effectiveness of minor lifestyle changes on diabetes management. Studies reveal that small adjustments, like incorporating more vegetables into meals or engaging in brief physical activities such as walking for 10 minutes after dinner, can lead to improved blood sugar levels and overall health (Michaelsen & Esch, 2023). These changes may seem insignificant individually, but collectively they reduce the risk of complications associated with diabetes and enhance quality of life.

The brain's ability to adapt, known as neuroplasticity, is another key factor in establishing tiny habits. When a new behavior is repeated frequently, neural pathways are strengthened, facilitating the transition from a deliberate act to an automatic response. For instance, if you start checking your blood sugar levels before each meal, your brain gradually adapts this behavior into a seamless part of your routine, reducing mental effort over time.

To make tiny habits effective in diabetes management, practical applications must be personalized. Identifying personal motivators is crucial. For some, the motivation might be the desire to stay healthy for their grandchildren, while for others it might be avoiding medical complications. Once motivators are identified, creating a supportive environment helps reinforce the habits. This can involve setting reminders, enlisting the support of family members, or rearranging one's living space to facilitate healthier choices. For example, replacing candy jars with bowls of fresh fruit makes it easier to choose a healthy snack.

Small actions are often underestimated, but they can have profound effects when applied consistently. By understanding the triggers that initiate behaviors and the rewards that follow, individuals can cultivate habits that improve their health without overwhelming themselves with drastic changes. For seniors managing diabetes, this is particularly beneficial, as it aligns with their need for practical, manageable strategies tailored to their lifestyle.

Behavioral psychology highlights the power of repetition in building habits. When actions are reliable triggered and rewarded, they engrain into routines. Health research substantiates that even minor dietary and physical activity adjustments can markedly improve diabetics' health, emphasizing the practicality of these approaches (Laborde et al., 2020). Neuroscience further elucidates that our brains are wired to adapt to repeated behaviors, solidifying them as habits over time.

Implementing tiny habits calls for identifying what motivates you. Is it spending more quality time with loved ones or reducing the risk of future health issues? Having clear motivators gives purpose to the small steps you take daily. Additionally, creating a conducive environment plays a significant role in the success of these tiny habits. Simple changes, like keeping healthy snacks within reach or setting alarms for medication, can significantly influence daily choices.

For effective management of diabetes through tiny habits, start small and stay consistent. Begin with one manageable change, like choosing whole grains over refined grains, and stick with it until it feels effortless. From there, you can gradually introduce other small changes, creating a cumulative effect that significantly enhances your health. Moreover, integrating physical activities in short, frequent bursts can be highly effective. Activities such as stretching during TV commercials or taking short walks after meals accumulate to provide substantial health benefits without requiring extensive time commitments.

Finally, involving supportive figures in your journey can amplify success.

Friends, family, and healthcare providers can offer encouragement and accountability, ensuring you stay on track with your habits. Share your goals with them and seek their support in maintaining these positive changes. For example, scheduling regular check-ins with a family member about your progress can keep you motivated and focused.

How Small Changes Lead to Big Results

Understanding the Power of Tiny Habits

In managing diabetes, especially for seniors, small lifestyle adjustments can lead to substantial health improvements. These minor changes often seem insignificant on their own, but when consistently practiced, they can transform one's health and well-being over time.

Transformation through Consistency: Regular engagement in small, health-oriented actions builds resilience and leads to transformative improvements. For example, one might start with simple habits such as walking for 10 minutes after each meal. These small increments of physical activity can gradually become a daily routine that significantly helps control blood sugar levels. Over time, these tiny habits create a foundation of regular exercise which builds physical resilience and improves overall health.

The power of consistency lies in its ability to make activities second nature. By repeating small actions each day, individuals can establish routines without feeling overwhelmed. For seniors, this approach can be especially beneficial as it avoids drastic disruptions to their established lifestyles. Additionally, consistent habits can provide a sense of accomplishment and stability, encouraging continued effort and progress.

Incremental Progress Stories: Real-life examples highlight the impact of minor dietary and exercise changes. Consider Joan, a 72-year-old grandmother who decided to replace her nightly dessert with a bowl of mixed berries. Initially, this seemed like a trivial change, but over six months, Joan noticed a notable improvement in her glucose levels. Paired with a five-minute stretching routine each morning, these small adjustments not only improved her health but also boosted her energy levels, allowing her to engage more actively with her grandchildren.

Another inspiring story is that of Tom, a retired teacher, who began substituting his afternoon coffee with herbal tea and added a short evening walk to his routine. These seemingly minor alterations helped Tom reduce his overall caffeine intake and increase physical activity, leading to better sleep patterns and a marked decrease in his fasting glucose readings. These stories underscore how small, manageable changes can lead to significant health benefits over time.

Compounding Effects: Linking small dietary changes with improved exercise routines amplifies health benefits and creates a healthier daily structure. For instance, combining a habit of choosing whole grains over refined grains with a daily 15-minute brisk walk can have a compounding effect. This synergy between diet and exercise not only enhances glucose metabolism but also improves cardiovascular health, reduces stress levels, and promotes weight management.

Studies show that even modest weight loss achieved through dietary changes and increased physical activity can result in significant health improvements (Galaviz et al., 2019). Seniors adopting small dietary modifications, like eating more leafy greens or reducing sugary snacks, alongside regular physical activity, may experience amplified benefits. Moreover, this compounded approach creates a structured daily routine, making it easier to adhere to both dietary and exercise goals.

Visualization Techniques: Practicing visualization and journaling can enhance commitment and motivate the adoption of new behaviors. Visualization involves imagining oneself successfully engaging in healthy habits, which can boost motivation and confidence. For seniors, visualizing themselves taking a leisurely walk in the park or enjoying a nutritious meal can make these activities more appealing and achievable.

Journaling complements visualization by providing a tangible way to track progress and reflect on successes and challenges. Writing down daily efforts, noting improvements in mood, energy levels, or glucose readings can reinforce positive behavior. For example, Mary, an 80-year-old retiree, started keeping a journal to log her daily walks and meals. Over time, she noticed patterns and was able to adjust her habits to better suit her needs. This practice kept her motivated and committed to maintaining her new healthy habits.

Combining visualization and journaling creates a powerful feedback loop. Imagining success makes the goal feel attainable, while documenting progress reinforces the behavior change. For caregivers and health professionals, encouraging seniors to visualize their health goals and keep a journal can be valuable tools in supporting long-term habit formation.

Implementing these tiny habits requires patience and persistence. Health professionals working with seniors should emphasize the importance of gradual changes and provide guidance on setting realistic goals. Caregivers can support their loved ones by celebrating small victories and encouraging consistency. By collectively focusing on incremental progress, it becomes easier to sustain these changes.

Examples of Effective Micro-Habits for Health

Integrating micro-habits into daily routines can significantly enhance health, particularly for seniors managing diabetes. By focusing on small, manageable changes, seniors can build sustainable habits that lead to long-term well-being.

Daily Actions

Incorporating simple daily actions can make a significant difference in overall health. For instance, drinking a glass of water first thing in the morning helps kickstart metabolism and keeps the body hydrated. This habit is easy to adopt and provides immediate benefits without requiring major lifestyle changes.

Standing up and moving around every hour is another effective micro-habit. Prolonged sitting can lead to various health issues, including poor blood circulation and increased risk of diabetes-related complications. Setting a timer as a reminder to stand up or walk around the house can break long periods of inactivity. This small action can improve blood flow and reduce the likelihood of developing further health problems.

Adding more fruit to meals is a straightforward way to enhance diet. Fruits are rich in essential vitamins, minerals, and fiber, which are crucial for regulating blood sugar levels. Replacing a sugary snack with a piece of fruit not only satisfies sweet cravings but also provides nutrients necessary for maintaining good health. Seniors can start by adding a serving of fruit to their breakfast or having it as an afternoon snack.

Mindful Eating

Mindful eating involves paying close attention to what and how you eat. One practical tip is to replace unhealthy snacks with healthier alternatives. For example, swapping chips for carrot sticks or nuts can significantly improve nutritional intake. These simple changes collectively contribute to better health by reducing the consumption of empty calories and boosting intake of essential nutrients.

Practicing awareness during meals is another powerful tool. This means eating slowly, savoring every bite, and paying attention to hunger and fullness cues. When individuals eat mindfully, they are more likely to appreciate their food and avoid overeating. A good practice is to set aside dedicated meal times without distractions like TV or phones, allowing full concentration on the eating experience.

Stress Management

Stress management is vital for emotional well-being and overall health, especially for seniors with diabetes. Small adjustments, such as deep breathing exercises before meals, can be highly beneficial. Deep breathing helps activate the body's relaxation response, lowering stress levels and improving digestion. Before each meal, taking a few moments to breathe deeply can set a calm tone, which aids in better digestion and nutrient absorption.

Daily gratitude reflections are another simple but effective practice. Taking a few minutes each day to reflect on positive aspects of life can improve mood and reduce stress. This can be done by keeping a gratitude journal or sharing thoughts with a loved one. Regularly acknowledging things one is thankful for fosters a positive mindset, which is crucial for emotional health.

Physical Movement

Incorporating short bursts of physical activity throughout the day is key to enhancing mobility. Simple activities, like standing while on the phone, can increase physical movement without requiring additional time commitment. This habit encourages more standing and less sitting, promoting better circulation and muscle engagement.

Taking the stairs instead of the elevator is another great example of a micro-habit that adds more activity to daily routines. For seniors, this might mean choosing to walk up one flight of stairs instead of riding the elevator or escalator for short distances. This small effort reinforces leg strength and cardiovascular health without needing a dedicated exercise session.

Seniors can also integrate other short activities, such as stretching or light yoga, into their daily routine. Stretching helps maintain flexibility and reduces muscle stiffness, while light yoga can improve balance and coordination. These activities can be done in short sessions, making them easy to fit into any schedule.

Guidelines for Adoption

To successfully incorporate these micro-habits, it's essential to start small and gradually build up. Consistency is key; therefore, picking one new habit at a time can prevent feeling overwhelmed. Using reminders, such as alarms or notes, can help reinforce these new habits until they become second nature.

For caregivers and family members, encouraging and participating in these habits can provide additional support. Shared activities, like going for a walk together or preparing healthy meals, not only reinforce the habits but also strengthen relationships and create a supportive environment.

Setting the Stage for Success

Creating a supportive environment for adopting and maintaining tiny habits is essential for effective diabetes management, particularly for seniors. The physical environment plays a crucial role in this process. By stocking healthy foods like fresh fruits, vegetables, lean proteins, and whole grains, you create an immediate option for healthier eating. Keeping these foods visible and easily accessible encourages their consumption over less healthy alternatives. Additionally, organizing spaces to promote physical activity can be very beneficial. For instance, setting up a small exercise corner with some light weights or resistance bands can act as a constant reminder to engage in physical activities. Simple changes like moving the TV remote away from the couch can encourage more walking.

The involvement of family and friends cannot be overstated in creating a conducive environment for habit formation. Social support systems provide accountability and shared motivation, both of which are critical for adopting new behaviors. Encouraging family members to participate in healthy activities like daily walks or preparing meals together can strengthen these new habits. Friends can also play a pivotal role by joining exercise classes designed for seniors or participating in community events that promote health. Regular check-ins with loved ones about progress can foster a sense of accomplishment and encourage further commitment to these habits.

Mental preparation is another key element in establishing and maintaining tiny habits. Positive affirmations can set the tone for success, while realistic expectations help avoid disappointment. Reflecting on past successes, no matter how small, builds confidence and motivation. Creating a vision board with images and words that represent goals and achievements can serve as a daily reminder of what you're working towards. Visualization techniques can also be helpful; imagining oneself successfully engaging in the desired behavior can make it feel more achievable and real.

Utilizing resources such as tools, checklists, reminders, and community programs can significantly aid in tracking progress and staying motivated. Checklists help keep tasks organized and ensure nothing is overlooked. Reminders, whether through phone alarms or sticky notes around the house, serve as constant prompts to engage in healthy behaviors. Community resources such as local diabetes support groups offer both educational materials and emotional support. These groups often have experienced individuals who can share practical tips and encouragement. Apps designed for diabetes management can also be highly useful. They often come with features like blood sugar tracking, meal planning guides, and reminders for medication, making it easier to stay on top of daily routines.

To delve deeper into each aspect, we start with the physical environment adjustments. These changes not only make healthy choices more accessible but also reduce the likelihood of reverting to old, unhealthy habits. For example, keeping a bowl of fruit on the kitchen counter makes it more likely that you'll reach for a piece of fruit instead of a sugary snack. Similarly, having a designated space for exercise, even if it's just a yoga mat and a few free weights, can serve as a visual cue to engage in physical activity.

Next, social support systems are vital for reinforcing new habits. When family members understand the importance of these small changes, they can provide much-needed encouragement and support. They can help ensure that the home environment is conducive to healthy living and join in on lifestyle changes, making it a shared endeavor rather than an individual challenge. Additionally, involving friends in your health journey provides an extra layer of accountability. Knowing that someone else is expecting you to show up for a walk or exercise class can be a powerful motivator.

Mental preparation involves developing a mindset that is open to change. Positive affirmations help build this mindset by focusing on what can be achieved rather than potential failures. Statements like "I am capable of managing my diabetes" or "Each small step I take improves my health" can replace negative thoughts and boost confidence. Setting realistic expectations is equally important. Understanding that change is gradual and celebrating small victories keeps you motivated and reduces feelings of overwhelm. Reflection on past successes also reinforces the belief that you can achieve your goals. Keeping a journal to document these successes can be a motivating tool to look back on during challenging times.

Lastly, the proper use of resources greatly enhances the ability to stick with new habits. Tools like checklists break down larger goals into manageable tasks, making it easier to focus on one thing at a time. Reminders ensure that these tasks are remembered and completed. Modern technology offers various resources through apps designed specifically for diabetes management. These apps provide functionalities like meal planning, glucose monitoring, and medication reminders. They also offer insights based on the data you input, helping you understand trends and make informed decisions. Community resources, such as local health workshops or online forums, offer additional support and information, providing opportunities to learn from others' experiences and share your own.

Final Thoughts

In this chapter, we've delved into how micro-habits can play a vital role in managing diabetes, particularly for seniors. By incorporating small, manageable changes into daily routines, such as drinking water in the morning or adding short walks after meals, substantial health improvements can be achieved over time. These tiny habits become second nature through consistent repetition, providing stability and a sense of accomplishment without overwhelming lifestyle disruptions. Real-life examples like Joan's switch to healthier dessert options and Tom's addition of herbal tea and evening walks highlight the profound impact of these minor adjustments on overall well-being.

Maintaining consistency in these small actions paves the way for lasting health benefits. The power of micro-habits lies in their simplicity and ease of integration into everyday life. Seniors can gain significant enhancements in blood sugar control, physical resilience, and emotional well-being by steadily building these habits. Support from family, friends, and caregivers further strengthens the adherence to these healthy routines, making the journey towards better diabetes management a shared, fulfilling endeavor. Remember, each small step taken with patience and persistence leads to big results in health and quality of life.

2

Mindful Eating: Small Changes, Big Impact

Mindful eating is a practice that can lead to significant health benefits, especially for seniors managing their blood sugar levels. Rather than making drastic changes, mindful eating focuses on small, intentional adjustments in eating habits. This approach encourages individuals to pay close attention to what and how much they eat while enjoying their food more fully. By adopting this mindset, seniors can make more thoughtful food choices, ultimately leading to better health outcomes and enhanced well-being.

In this chapter, you will explore various techniques to help implement mindful eating practices. The focus will be on understanding portion control, which is crucial in maintaining balanced diets and preventing overconsumption. Practical tips such as measuring food portions accurately and using visual cues will be discussed to make mindful eating easier to practice. Additionally, strategies for serving food in ways that support smaller portions and gradual reduction methods will be shared. These insights aim to empower seniors, caregivers, and health professionals with actionable steps to promote healthier eating habits and improve blood sugar management through mindful eating.

Portion Control Techniques

Managing portion sizes is a pivotal strategy for seniors looking to control their blood sugar levels and improve overall health. This section aims to provide clear and actionable advice on how to manage portions effectively to help maintain a balanced diet.

Understanding Portion Sizes

A fundamental aspect of mindful eating is understanding what constitutes a sensible portion size for various food groups. For instance, a serving of carbohydrates like pasta or rice should be about the size of your fist or roughly half a cup cooked. Protein servings, such as chicken or fish, should be about the size of your palm or approximately three ounces. Vegetables are an essential part of a balanced diet, and it's generally beneficial to fill half your plate with non-starchy vegetables like broccoli, spinach, or bell peppers. Fruit servings should be limited to one small piece like an apple or a half-cup of chopped fruit. Dairy products, which are important for bone health, should be kept to one cup of milk or yogurt. Understanding these basic portion sizes can make it easier to balance your diet without overindulging in any particular food group.

Measuring and Serving Practice

Accurately measuring food portions can significantly aid in maintaining healthy portion sizes. Tools like measuring cups and kitchen scales are invaluable for this purpose. When you use a measuring cup to portion out your oatmeal in the morning or measure a serving of rice for dinner, you gain a clearer understanding of how much you are actually consuming. Visual cues can also be helpful. For example, if you don't have a measuring tool handy, remember that a serving of meat should be about the size of a deck of cards, while a serving of cheese can be compared to the size of four dice stacked together.

For liquids, measuring spoons help ensure you are not inadvertently adding more calories than intended, particularly with items like cooking oils and dressings. Additionally, pre-portioning snacks into small containers can prevent overeating. Instead of eating directly from a large bag of nuts or chips, distribute them into single-serving containers. This practice will help you become more aware of the quantity you are consuming and reduce the likelihood of exceeding recommended portion sizes.

Mindful Serving Practices

How food is served can influence your eating habits significantly. Family-style serving, where dishes are placed on the table for everyone to serve themselves, often leads to larger portions and second helpings. Instead, try serving individual portions directly onto plates before bringing them to the table. This approach helps in controlling the amount of food consumed by limiting the temptation to take extra servings.

Another mindful practice is to use smaller plates and bowls. Smaller dishes make portions appear larger, tricking your brain into feeling satisfied with less food. Research shows that people tend to eat less when they use smaller plates because it gives the illusion of a fuller plate, which can psychologically lead to improved satiety. Additionally, avoid eating straight from packages, as it becomes difficult to track how much you've eaten. By placing food onto a plate or bowl, you create a physical limit to your portions.

Gradual Portion Reduction

Making drastic changes to portion sizes can be overwhelming and hard to sustain. A more effective approach is to gradually reduce portion sizes. Start by setting small, achievable goals, such as reducing your portion of pasta by one tablespoon each week until you reach the recommended half-cup serving. This incremental reduction allows your body and mind to adjust to the smaller portions without feeling deprived.

Weekly goals can extend to other areas of your diet as well. For example, if you're used to having two slices of bread with your sandwich, try using just one slice and substituting the rest with leafy greens or another vegetable. Similarly, if your usual dessert is a large bowl of ice cream, consider reducing the portion slightly each week while increasing the amount of fresh fruit you include as a topping. These small adjustments accumulate over time, leading to significant improvements in managing calorie intake and blood sugar levels.

Involving family members or caregivers in this process can provide additional support and accountability. Discuss your goals with them and ask for their assistance in preparing meals that align with your portion control objectives. Engaging in these practices together can create a supportive environment that makes it easier to stick to your new habits.

Identifying Healthy Food Swaps

Understanding Food Labels: Knowing how to read food labels is essential for making healthier food choices, especially for managing diabetes. Food labels provide crucial information about the nutritional content and ingredients of packaged foods. Start by looking at the serving size because all the nutritional information on the label is based on this. Next, check the calories per serving, which will help you manage your calorie intake. Pay attention to macronutrients like fats, carbohydrates, and proteins to ensure they align with your dietary goals. Also, look for key nutrients such as fiber, vitamins, and minerals that are beneficial for your health.

The ingredient list is equally important. Ingredients are listed in descending order by weight, so the first few make up the bulk of the product. Avoid items with lengthy lists of unfamiliar or overly processed ingredients. Be particularly wary of additives and preservatives; opt for products with minimal or no additives. Lastly, check for allergens and be mindful of sodium and sugar content as excessive amounts can contribute to health issues.

Simple Swaps for Common Foods: Making small changes to everyday food choices can have a big impact on managing diabetes. For instance, swapping white bread for whole-grain options adds more fiber to your diet, which helps control blood sugar levels. Instead of sugary cereals, opt for oatmeal or high-fiber cereals. Replace regular pasta with whole-wheat or vegetable-based alternatives. These swaps not only improve nutrient intake but also help stabilize blood sugar levels.

Consider switching from full-fat dairy products to low-fat or non-fat versions. Choose lean meats like chicken or turkey over fatty cuts of beef and pork. When it comes to snacks, replace chips and cookies with fruits, nuts, or yogurt. These simple swaps can make a significant difference in your overall health and diabetes management.

The Power of Flavor: Eating healthy doesn't mean sacrificing flavor. You can enhance the taste of your meals using herbs, spices, and different cooking methods. Herbs like basil, cilantro, and dill add freshness and aroma to dishes without adding calories or sodium. Spices like cinnamon, turmeric, and cumin not only enhance flavor but also offer health benefits. For example, cinnamon has been shown to help lower blood sugar levels.

Experiment with different cooking methods like grilling, roasting, and steaming to bring out the natural flavors of foods. Marinating meats and vegetables before cooking can also add depth of flavor. Using citrus juices, vinegar, and olive oil as dressings can make salads more enjoyable. By focusing on flavor, you can make healthy eating both delicious and satisfying.

Creating a Swaps List: Once you've identified healthier food options, it's helpful to create a personalized swaps list. This list can serve as a quick reference when grocery shopping or planning meals. Write down your favorite unhealthy foods and find healthier alternatives for each. For example, if you love ice cream, try frozen yogurt or a smoothie made with frozen fruits and Greek yogurt instead.

Keep your swaps list handy in the kitchen and update it regularly as you discover new healthy options. Involve family members and caregivers in creating and maintaining the list to ensure everyone is on board with the healthier choices. This collaborative approach can make it easier to integrate these swaps into daily meals sustainably.

Eating Slowly and Savoring Meals

The Science of Slow Eating

Eating slowly and mindfully can have a profound impact on digestion and blood sugar control, which is particularly important for seniors managing diabetes. When we eat too quickly, our bodies do not have sufficient time to signal that we're full, leading to overeating. Research shows that it takes about 20 minutes for the brain to receive signals from the stomach that it's full. By slowing down, we allow this natural process to occur, helping to prevent overconsumption and aiding in the regulation of blood sugar levels (Welp, 2023).

Additionally, thorough chewing enhances nutrient absorption and digestion. Salivary enzymes begin breaking down food in the mouth, setting the stage for more efficient digestion throughout the gastrointestinal tract. Moreover, slower eating helps reduce the workload on the digestive system, potentially alleviating common issues such as indigestion and bloating.

Techniques to Slow Down

Incorporating slow eating into daily routines doesn't require drastic changes but rather small, mindful adjustments. One practical technique is to put utensils down between bites. This simple action forces a pause, giving you time to chew thoroughly and savor each bite, fostering a more relaxed eating pace. Another effective method is taking deep breaths between bites. This practice not only slows down your eating but also helps engage the parasympathetic nervous system, which supports digestion and reduces stress (Cherpak, 2019).

Another approach is to listen to guided meditation or breathwork exercises before meals. These practices shift your body towards a rest-and-digest state, promoting mindfulness and enhancing the overall eating experience. Regularly using a hunger scale before and after meals can also be beneficial. By rating your hunger and fullness on a scale from one to ten, you develop a better understanding of your body's signals, encouraging you to stop eating when you're comfortably satisfied instead of overly full.

Savoring Flavors

One of the joys of mindful eating is the opportunity to fully engage with the sensory experiences of food. Savoring flavors means paying close attention to the tastes, textures, and aromas of what you're eating. This practice not only makes meals more enjoyable but also helps reduce the urge to overeat by increasing satisfaction and satiety.

Engaging all your senses while eating can enhance the pleasure derived from food. Notice the vibrant colors on your plate, inhale the rich aromas, and feel the different textures in your mouth. By focusing on these sensory details, you make each meal an event, rather than a rushed necessity. For example, take a small piece of dark chocolate and let it melt in your mouth, appreciating its bitterness and texture. Similarly, sucking on a fresh lemon half can help you appreciate its sourness and stimulate digestive secretions.

Creating Mindful Eating Rituals

Developing mindful eating rituals can significantly enhance the eating experience and promote better health outcomes. A key aspect of mindful eating is creating an environment free from distractions, allowing you to focus entirely on the act of eating. This might involve turning off electronic devices, clearing the table of unrelated items, and perhaps lighting a candle to create a calm atmosphere (Cherpak, 2019).

Sharing meals with family or friends can also foster mindfulness. Conversation during meals encourages slower eating and allows you to enjoy both your food and the company around you. Make it a practice to express gratitude for your meal before eating. This simple ritual can shift your mindset, making you more aware and appreciative of the food you are about to consume.

Moreover, establishing routines, such as eating at the same times each day and having dedicated meal areas, can further reinforce mindful eating habits. Over time, these small actions build a foundation for healthier eating patterns, contributing to better digestion and blood sugar control.

Practical Tips for Caregivers and Health Professionals

Caregivers and health professionals play a crucial role in supporting seniors' efforts to adopt mindful eating practices. Offering practical advice and demonstrating techniques can empower seniors to make positive changes. Encourage them to start with small, manageable steps such as putting down utensils between bites or spending a few moments to breathe deeply before meals.

Providing visual cues or reminders can also be helpful. For instance, placing a note on the table that says "slow down" can serve as a gentle reminder to eat more mindfully. Additionally, caregivers can model mindful eating behaviors during shared meals, reinforcing the practice through example.

Health professionals should consider integrating discussions about mindful eating into routine care. Discussing the benefits and providing resources like guided meditations or instructional videos can greatly aid in the adoption of these practices. Tailored advice that aligns with the senior's lifestyle and preferences will likely yield the best results.

Conclusion

Mindful eating is a powerful tool for improving digestion and blood sugar control, especially for seniors managing diabetes. By understanding the science behind slow eating, practicing techniques to eat more mindfully, savoring the flavors and sensory experiences of food, and creating supportive rituals, seniors can make lasting positive changes to their eating habits.

Employing these strategies in daily routines requires consistent effort but offers significant rewards in terms of health and well-being. Caregivers and health professionals can support this journey by providing guidance, encouragement, and resources tailored to the needs of seniors.

Reading and Understanding Nutrition Labels

Understanding nutrition labels is crucial for making informed food choices, especially for seniors who need to manage their blood sugar levels. This section provides simple guidelines and practical advice to help seniors interpret these labels effectively.

Key Components of Nutrition Labels

Nutrition labels can seem overwhelming, but understanding key components can simplify the process.

Serving Size: The serving size is listed at the top of the nutrition label. This information is vital as all nutritional values on the label are based on this serving. For example, if the serving size is one cup and you consume two cups, you're getting twice the calories, fat, and other nutrients listed.

Calories: Calories are a measure of energy. Knowing the calorie content helps in choosing foods that fit within your daily caloric needs. Seniors should be aware that different foods have varying calorie densities; for instance, nuts have more calories per gram compared to vegetables.

Nutrients to Focus On: Pay attention to key nutrients such as total fat, cholesterol, sodium, total carbohydrates (including dietary fiber and sugars), protein, vitamins, and minerals. Understanding these elements helps in assessing the healthfulness of foods. Excessive intake of fats, cholesterol, and sodium can contribute to chronic diseases, making it crucial to monitor these nutrients.

Identifying Hidden Sugars

Hidden sugars can pose a significant problem, especially for those managing diabetes. Food manufacturers often add various forms of sugar to enhance flavor, which might not always be obvious on the labels.

Sugar isn't always labeled simply as 'sugar.' It can appear under many names, including sucrose, high-fructose corn syrup, dextrose, and agave nectar, among others. Recognizing these names can help avoid high-sugar products. When checking the ingredient list, look out for terms ending in "-ose," as they signify types of sugar.

To avoid these hidden sugars, it's helpful to reference the "added sugars" section on the nutrition label. As of January 2021, added sugars must be explicitly listed, making it easier to differentiate between naturally occurring sugars and those added during processing (Reading Food Labels | ADA, n.d.). Reducing intake of added sugars can significantly help in managing blood sugar levels.

Understanding Ingredients Lists

The ingredients list can tell you a lot about what you're consuming. Ingredients are listed in order of quantity used in the product, from highest to lowest.

Shorter ingredient lists with recognizable items are generally better choices. For instance, a loaf of whole-grain bread should include ingredients like whole wheat flour, water, yeast, and salt. Avoid products with long lists of unrecognizable chemicals and additives, as they often indicate highly processed foods.

When selecting products, also ensure the primary ingredients are whole foods. For example, in whole grain products, look for "100% whole wheat flour" rather than just "wheat flour," which may be refined and less nutritious.

Making Quick Decisions

Shopping for healthy foods doesn't have to be time-consuming. Here are some quick tips for efficiently assessing nutrition labels:

Carry a List: Having a list of key nutrients to check, such as calories, total fat, sodium, and added sugars, can save time. Before heading to the store, write down or print a small card listing these critical points.

Use Percent Daily Values (%DV): The %DV shows how much a nutrient in a serving of food contributes to your daily diet. Aim for lower percentages of saturated fats, sodium, and sugars, and higher percentages of fibers, vitamins, and minerals. A general rule of thumb is 5% DV or less is low, and 20% DV or more is high for any nutrient.

Scan for Keywords: Quickly scan the product's front packaging for keywords related to its health benefits or pitfalls. Ignore marketing claims like "natural" or "low-fat" and instead focus on verifiable details like "whole grain" or "no added sugars."

Check Sodium Content: Sodium can sneak into almost everything, from soups to sauces. Compare labels to choose options with lower sodium content.

A handy tip is to ensure milligrams of sodium don't exceed the number of calories per serving, keeping your intake balanced (4 Tips for Reading Food Labels That Will Change the Way You Shop, 2016).

Summary and Reflections

In this chapter, we've delved into the concept of mindful eating and its significant impact on controlling blood sugar levels for seniors. By understanding proper portion sizes and using practical tools like measuring cups and kitchen scales, you can make more informed decisions about your daily food intake. Implementing strategies such as using smaller plates, pre-portioning snacks, and gradually reducing portion sizes can help you maintain a balanced diet without feeling deprived. These small yet powerful changes in your eating habits can contribute to better blood sugar management and overall health.

Remember, mindful eating goes beyond just the physical aspects; it also involves savoring each bite and being fully present during meals. Techniques like putting down utensils between bites and taking deep breaths can slow down your eating pace, enhancing digestion and satisfaction. Enlisting support from family members and caregivers can make this journey easier and more enjoyable. By adopting these mindful eating practices, you can effectively manage your blood sugar levels and improve your quality of life.

3

Getting Active: Easy Exercises for Seniors

Getting active through simple exercises can be a game-changer for seniors managing diabetes. Incorporating physical activity into daily routines not only helps regulate blood sugar levels but also brings a host of other health benefits. This chapter aims to inspire and guide you with easy-to-follow exercises that fit seamlessly into your everyday life. These activities are designed to be gentle yet effective, making them suitable for those new to exercise or who may have mobility issues.

In this chapter, you'll discover a variety of home-based exercises tailored to seniors. We will explore chair exercises, gentle stretching routines, resistance band workouts, and balance exercises—all of which can significantly improve your strength, flexibility, and overall well-being. Whether you're looking to boost your energy, enhance your mood, or simply stay more active, these exercises offer practical and enjoyable ways to achieve your health goals. By the end of this chapter, you'll be equipped with the knowledge and motivation to make physical activity an integral part of your daily routine.

Benefits of Regular Exercise

Regular exercise is a cornerstone of effective diabetes management and overall well-being, especially for seniors. Engaging in physical activities can significantly enhance insulin sensitivity, which helps maintain stable blood sugar levels. Insulin sensitivity refers to how effectively your body uses insulin to lower blood sugar. When you exercise, your muscles take up more glucose from your bloodstream, reducing the amount of insulin needed to manage your blood sugar. This is particularly helpful for those with type 2 diabetes or prediabetes, as it combats insulin resistance – a condition where cells in your muscles, fat, and liver don't respond well to insulin.

Physical activity also has profound effects on mental health. Exercise releases endorphins, often referred to as 'feel-good hormones'. These chemicals interact with receptors in your brain that reduce your perception of pain and trigger positive feelings, similar to those produced by morphine. For many seniors, this means improved mood, reduced anxiety, and even alleviation of mild depression symptoms. It's not just about feeling happier; these mood-boosting benefits can translate into increased motivation to stick with an exercise regimen, creating a positive feedback loop.

Additionally, regular movement can battle fatigue and enhance vitality, making daily tasks less daunting. Many seniors struggle with low energy levels, but frequent physical activity can help address this issue. It may seem counterintuitive, but expending energy through exercise actually generates more energy. One reason is that physical activity improves cardiovascular efficiency, meaning your heart and lungs work better to supply oxygen and nutrients to tissues. This leads to an increase in stamina and reduces the likelihood of feeling worn out after minimal exertion.

Better sleep quality is another significant benefit of routine exercise. Many older adults experience sleep disturbances, from difficulty falling asleep to waking up frequently during the night. Exercise helps regulate your body's internal clock or circadian rhythm, ensuring you feel sleepy at the right time and wake up feeling refreshed. Physical activity also increases the time you spend in deep sleep, which is the most restorative phase of sleep. Deep sleep boosts immune function, supports cardiac health, and controls stress and anxiety.

The positive impact of regular exercise extends to heart health, significantly reducing factors associated with heart disease and stroke. Heart disease is a leading cause of death among seniors, and diabetes only heightens this risk. However, routine physical activity can mitigate these risks by improving circulatory health, lowering blood pressure, and reducing bad cholesterol levels. Exercise fosters the growth of new blood vessels, improves heart muscle function, and enhances overall blood flow, ensuring that organs and tissues receive adequate oxygen and nutrients.

Even light exercises can yield substantial benefits. For instance, simple activities such as brisk walking, gardening, or light aerobic sessions can be incredibly effective. The key is consistency rather than intensity. Seniors do not need to engage in strenuous workouts to reap the rewards. In fact, low-intensity, high-frequency exercises might be safer and more sustainable, reducing the risk of injury while keeping the body active.

Moreover, exercise aids in weight management, which is crucial for controlling diabetes. Excess weight, particularly around the abdomen, is a major factor in the development of type 2 diabetes because it increases insulin resistance. Regular physical activity helps burn calories and build muscle mass, which raises your metabolic rate. More muscle mass means you'll burn more calories even at rest, contributing to long-term weight control.

Besides its physical benefits, engaging in regular exercise provides invaluable social interaction opportunities. Whether it's joining a walking group or participating in community fitness classes, these activities encourage socialization and combat loneliness, a common issue among seniors. Social engagement, coupled with physical activity, has been shown to improve mental health outcomes significantly.

Starting an exercise routine doesn't require a gym membership or expensive equipment. Simple home-based exercises can be equally effective. Chair exercises, for example, are perfect for individuals with mobility issues. These low-impact exercises focus on strength and flexibility and can be performed while sitting or standing next to a chair for support.

Simple Home-Based Exercises

Incorporating physical activity into daily routines is essential for seniors managing diabetes and seeking to improve their overall health. Practical exercise routines that can be performed at home without needing a gym offer a convenient way to stay active. Here, we discuss accessible exercises tailored for seniors, including chair exercises, gentle stretching, resistance band workouts, and balance exercises.

Chair Exercises

Chair exercises support maintaining fitness levels without requiring much space or equipment. These exercises are particularly beneficial for seniors with limited mobility or those who find it challenging to perform standing exercises. Simple movements such as leg lifts and arm raises can significantly enhance muscle strength and flexibility.

For example, knee extensions are an effective chair exercise. To perform knee extensions:

1. Sit in a sturdy chair with your feet flat on the floor and back straight.
2. Slowly extend your right leg until it's parallel to the ground.
3. Hold this position for a couple of seconds before lowering your leg back down.
4. Repeat for 10–15 reps and switch to the left leg.

Seated marches can also boost cardiovascular health and aid hip flexor mobility. The steps for seated marches are:

1. Sit upright with your feet flat on the floor.
2. Lift your right knee toward your chest.
3. Lower your right knee and lift your left knee in the same motion.
4. Alternate between legs for 1–2 minutes, maintaining smooth and controlled movements.

Gentle Stretching

Gentle stretching exercises play a crucial role in improving flexibility and reducing stiffness, which is vital for daily routines. Stretching helps keep muscles supple and joints flexible, making everyday movements easier and more comfortable.

Stretching exercises like shoulder circles are simple yet effective. Here's how to do shoulder circles:

1. Sit or stand with your feet shoulder-width apart.

2. Slowly roll your shoulders forward in a circular motion for about 20 seconds.
3. Reverse the direction and roll your shoulders backward for another 20 seconds.

Hamstring stretches are also beneficial for flexibility. Follow these steps for hamstring stretches while seated:

1. Sit on the edge of a chair with one foot flat on the floor and the other leg extended straight out in front, heel touching the floor.
2. Gently lean forward from your hips, keeping your back straight, until you feel a stretch in the back of your thigh.
3. Hold the stretch for 15-30 seconds and then switch legs.

Resistance Band Workouts

Resistance band workouts provide low-impact strength training, which is beneficial for glucose metabolism. Resistance bands are portable, affordable, and can easily be adjusted to accommodate different strength levels. They help build muscle strength, which is crucial for managing diabetes and enhancing overall physical health.

A basic resistance band workout to try is the seated bicep curl. Here's how to perform it:

1. Sit on a chair with your feet flat on the floor.
2. Hold the resistance band handles, with the center of the band secured under your feet.
3. Keep your elbows close to your sides and pull the handles toward your shoulders.
4. Slowly lower the handles back to the starting position.
5. Perform 10-15 reps and rest before repeating.

Another effective resistance band exercise is the standing leg press:

1. Stand with one end of the resistance band secured around a sturdy object and the other end looped around your ankle.
2. Face away from the anchored end and stand on one leg for balance.
3. Extend your leg with the band, pushing against the resistance.
4. Return to the starting position and repeat 10-15 times before switching legs.

Balance Exercises

Balance exercises are paramount for enhancing stability and preventing falls, which are common concerns among seniors. Improving balance not only aids in performing daily activities but also boosts confidence and independence.

One simple balance exercise is the single-leg stance. Here's how to practice it safely:

1. Stand behind a sturdy chair, holding onto it for support.
2. Lift one foot off the ground and balance on the other leg.
3. Hold this position for as long as possible, aiming for 30 seconds.
4. Switch to the other leg and repeat.
5. Gradually reduce reliance on the chair as balance improves.

Heel-to-toe walking is another effective balance exercise. Follow these steps:

1. Walk in a straight line, placing one foot directly in front of the other, so the heel of one foot touches the toes of the opposite foot.
2. Focus on a fixed point ahead to maintain balance.
3. Take 20 steps, turn around, and walk back.

Regular practice of these exercises can lead to noticeable improvements in balance, helping prevent falls and related injuries.

Conclusion

Walking as a Powerful Habit

Walking is one of the simplest and most effective exercises that seniors can easily incorporate into their daily lives. It demands no special equipment, making it accessible for nearly everyone. Whether in a local park, around the neighborhood, or even indoors at a shopping mall, walking is an adaptable activity suited to various environments.

Accessibility is a key advantage of walking. Unlike gym-based activities that may require memberships, expensive machines, or specialized gear, walking simply necessitates a comfortable pair of shoes. This minimalistic approach not only reduces barriers but also promotes inclusivity, ensuring that more seniors can participate without feeling daunted by financial or logistical constraints.

To make walking a regular part of daily life, setting specific times for walks can be immensely beneficial. Consistency helps build habits, and designating certain times of the day for walking turns it into a routine. For instance, taking a walk after breakfast or before dinner can become a cherished part of the day, providing structure and predictability. This planned approach helps ensure that daily walks are not just occasional activities but rather integral components of one's lifestyle.

Joining walking groups adds another layer of motivation and enjoyment to this simple exercise. Social interaction has profound benefits for mental health, combating feelings of loneliness and isolation which many seniors might experience. Walking with a group or even a single walking buddy provides mutual encouragement and makes the activity more enjoyable. It's easier to look forward to walking when it's linked to pleasant conversations and shared experiences. Moreover, group walks instill a sense of accountability, as participants are less likely to skip a session if others are expecting them.

Tracking progress is an essential aspect of maintaining motivation and achieving fitness goals. Pedometers and smartphone apps serve as valuable tools in this regard. By monitoring steps taken, distance covered, or calories burned, these devices provide tangible evidence of one's efforts and improvements. Many apps allow users to set personalized goals, such as a certain number of steps per day or total distances each week. Visual representations like graphs and charts make it easy to see progress over time, adding a rewarding dimension to the exercise. Specific apps designed for seniors, such as Pacer or Map My Walk, offer user-friendly interfaces and features tailored to meet older adults' needs, making tracking both straightforward and encouraging (Felberbaum et al., 2023).

In addition to tracking steps and distances, these applications often come with additional functionalities such as reminders to walk, guided audio workouts, and social features that let users connect with friends or join online communities. These features cater to different preferences and needs, allowing seniors to select what works best for them.

Another significant benefit of utilizing technology in walking is the ability to log how one feels after each walk. This practice helps identify patterns and symptoms, which can be crucial for adjusting routines to optimize health benefits. For example, if a senior notices they feel particularly energetic and positive after a morning walk, they might prioritize this time of day for future walks.

Joining walking groups and using technology to monitor progress isn't just about physical health; it's equally about enhancing the overall quality of life. Regular interaction with peers through walking groups can foster meaningful relationships, providing emotional support and building a stronger community. This sense of belonging and connection is vital for mental well-being.

On the practical side, those concerned about staying motivated can find substantial support from walking technologies. Features such as milestone celebrations and virtual rewards offer external encouragement, recognizing individual achievements in a fun and engaging way. This gamification element keeps the activity light-hearted and something to look forward to.

When beginning a new walking routine, it's helpful to start slowly and increase intensity gradually. Overdoing it can lead to fatigue or injury, which may discourage continued participation. Apps that provide beginner-friendly programs can guide seniors in pacing themselves appropriately. They can remind users to warm up before starting, cool down after finishing, and stay hydrated throughout the walk—essential practices for maintaining safety and maximizing benefits.

For seniors with mobility issues, there are adaptations and alternatives within these technologies. Certain apps offer seated exercises or other low-impact activities that can be tracked similarly to walking. This adaptability ensures that even those unable to walk long distances can still engage in beneficial physical activity.

It's clear that integrating walking into daily routines provides numerous advantages. The lack of required equipment removes common barriers, while joining walking groups enhances motivation through social interaction. Setting specific walking times and using technology to track progress further supports these efforts by creating consistency and measurable accomplishments.

Using Technology to Track Progress

Incorporating technology into fitness routines can greatly benefit seniors by providing them with tools to monitor their physical activity and set health goals. One of the most accessible forms of technology to assist in this endeavor is wearable devices. Fitness trackers, such as Fitbit or Garmin, are designed to measure steps taken, heart rate, and calories burned. These devices offer real-time feedback and can motivate seniors to stay active by setting daily step goals or reminding them to move throughout the day. Moreover, many fitness trackers come equipped with features that help monitor sleep patterns, which is crucial for overall health.

The integration of health and fitness apps can further enhance the experience of using these wearable devices. Apps like MyFitnessPal, Argus, and Apple Health provide comprehensive tracking capabilities. They allow users to log various types of exercise, track nutritional intake, and set personalized fitness goals. These apps often sync with wearable devices, offering a seamless way to monitor progress over time. (Kononova et al., 2019) highlight the importance of goal setting and self-monitoring in promoting physical activity among older adults. By simplifying the process of recording and analyzing exercise data, these apps make it easier for seniors to understand their activity levels and identify areas for improvement.

For seniors who prefer structured exercise routines, online platforms offer a wealth of guided workouts that cater to all fitness levels. Websites and apps like SilverSneakers, YouTube, and Peloton provide access to a wide range of exercise classes—from gentle yoga and chair exercises to more vigorous aerobics—all from the comfort of home. This not only adds variety to their workout regimen but also ensures consistency. Engaging with these resources can be particularly beneficial for those who may have difficulty attending in-person classes. Online classes often come with professional instructors who demonstrate proper form and technique, reducing the risk of injury and improving the effectiveness of each workout.

Another significant aspect of incorporating technology into fitness routines is involving family members. Family support can play a critical role in maintaining motivation and accountability. Seniors can share their progress through apps or social media platforms, receiving encouragement and advice from loved ones. This can foster a sense of connection and make the fitness journey more enjoyable. Families can also participate in virtual fitness challenges together or track each other's progress, creating a supportive environment that encourages everyone to stay active. This collective approach not only strengthens familial bonds but also promotes long-term adherence to physical activity.

Exploring wearable devices such as fitness trackers is a practical first step for seniors looking to monitor their physical activity. These devices are user-friendly and provide valuable insights into daily movement patterns. For instance, a senior might discover that they are more active in the mornings and can plan their activities accordingly. Some fitness trackers also offer reminders to stand up and move if they detect prolonged periods of inactivity, which can be especially useful for those at risk of becoming too sedentary.

Health and fitness apps complement these wearable devices by offering detailed analytics and goal-setting features. Many apps are designed with ease of use in mind, featuring large text, intuitive interfaces, and customizable alerts. They can track a wide range of metrics, from cardiovascular fitness and strength training to flexibility and mindfulness practices. Seniors can easily log their food intake, monitor hydration levels, and even receive tips on healthy recipes and meal planning. The ability to visualize progress through charts and summaries can be incredibly motivating, helping seniors see the tangible benefits of their efforts.

Utilizing online fitness platforms can bring a new dimension to at-home workouts. These platforms provide access to certified trainers and tailored programs that address the specific needs of older adults. For example, seniors can choose low-impact workouts that focus on joint mobility and balance, which are crucial for preventing falls and maintaining independence. Participating in live-streamed classes or pre-recorded sessions offers flexibility, allowing seniors to fit exercise into their schedules without leaving home. Additionally, some platforms offer community features where users can interact with others, share experiences, and gain additional support.

Engaging family members in the fitness journey is another powerful strategy. When seniors involve their loved ones, they create an environment of mutual support and shared goals. Family members can participate in joint exercise sessions, whether it's a walk in the park, a home yoga class, or a virtual dance party. Sharing achievements and milestones through group chats or dedicated fitness apps can inspire friendly competition and collective celebration of progress. This collaborative approach helps maintain enthusiasm and commitment, making physical activity a fun and integral part of daily life.

Bringing It All Together

Incorporating light physical activities into daily routines can have a profound impact on managing diabetes and enhancing overall health for seniors. This chapter has highlighted the numerous benefits of regular exercise, from improving insulin sensitivity and cardiovascular health to boosting mental well-being and sleep quality. By engaging in simple movements like chair exercises, gentle stretching, resistance band workouts, and balance exercises, seniors can experience significant improvements in their energy levels, flexibility, and stability. These activities not only aid in weight management but also offer social interaction opportunities that combat loneliness and foster a sense of community.

Remember, consistency is key when it comes to reaping the rewards of physical activity. Whether it's walking regularly, joining a group exercise class, or using technology to track progress, establishing a routine and sticking with it can lead to lasting positive changes. The goal isn't to perform strenuous workouts but rather to find enjoyable and sustainable ways to stay active. By integrating these practical exercise routines into your daily life, you can take meaningful steps towards better diabetes management and an improved quality of life.

4

Mastering Stress: Mindfulness and Relaxation

astering stress is a vital aspect of managing diabetes and maintaining overall well-being. Mindfulness and relaxation techniques play an essential role in reducing stress, allowing seniors to live a calmer and healthier life. For seniors with diabetes, learning how to stay present without judgment can help alleviate the pressures of managing this chronic condition. The ability to focus on the current moment not only fosters emotional peace but also enhances clarity, making everyday challenges more manageable.

In this chapter, we'll explore various strategies to integrate mindfulness and relaxation into daily routines. We'll start by delving into the principles of mindfulness meditation, highlighting its benefits for emotional resilience and self-awareness. You'll find practical tips for practicing mindfulness, from sitting quietly and focusing on your breath to incorporating mindful eating and walking into your daily activities. We will also cover deep breathing exercises like the 4-7-8 technique, which can be employed during stressful moments to promote calmness and stabilize blood sugar levels. Lastly, you'll learn how to create a supportive environment at home that minimizes stress and enhances relaxation. Through these approaches, you and your caregivers can build a robust framework to not only manage diabetes effectively but also improve your overall quality of life.

Basics of Mindfulness Meditation

Mindfulness meditation is an invaluable tool for managing stress and maintaining emotional well-being, especially for seniors dealing with diabetes. Understanding the fundamental principles of mindfulness and its benefits can empower older adults to lead more relaxed, healthier lives.

Mindfulness is the practice of being present in the moment without judgment. It involves focusing on the current experience rather than dwelling on past events or worrying about the future. This mental shift allows individuals to fully engage with their surroundings and sensations, fostering a sense of peace and clarity. For seniors, this focused attention can significantly reduce anxiety linked to reminiscing about past regrets or fretting over future uncertainties.

One of the most profound benefits of mindfulness is its ability to improve emotional resilience. Emotional resilience refers to the capacity to recover quickly from difficulties. Mindfulness helps by encouraging a non-reactive awareness of one's thoughts and emotions. For seniors managing diabetes, this increased resilience means they can handle stressors related to their condition with calmness and clarity. When faced with a high blood sugar reading or other diabetes-related challenges, a mindful approach allows for thoughtful responses rather than panic or frustration.

Practicing mindfulness also enhances self-awareness. This heightened awareness enables seniors to recognize when they are beginning to feel stressed and identify specific triggers. Being able to pinpoint these triggers is crucial because it allows for proactive stress management. For example, if a senior notices that checking blood sugar levels causes anxiety, they can incorporate calming mindfulness techniques before testing to mitigate this stress.

In addition to reducing stress and improving emotional resilience, mindfulness meditation offers several other health benefits linked to diabetes management. Studies have shown that regular mindfulness practice can lower blood pressure, which is particularly beneficial for seniors who often experience hypertension. Lower blood pressure reduces the risk of heart disease and stroke, common complications of diabetes, thereby contributing to overall well-being.

Moreover, mindfulness meditation has been found to enhance cognitive functioning, which includes memory and attention span. As people age, cognitive decline becomes a concern, and for those with diabetes, maintaining mental sharpness is vital. Meditation techniques such as mindful breathing or body scans help seniors stay mentally engaged and alert. This improved cognitive function supports better decision-making and adherence to diabetes management plans.

For seniors seeking to cultivate mindfulness in their daily lives, there are simple, practical steps to get started. Begin by dedicating a few minutes each day to sit quietly and focus on your breath. Notice the sensation of the air entering and leaving your nostrils. If your mind wanders, gently bring your attention back to your breath. This practice can be done anywhere and at any time, making it easily accessible.

Incorporating mindfulness into everyday routines can further enhance its benefits. Seniors can practice mindful eating by paying close attention to the taste, texture, and aroma of their food. This not only makes meals more enjoyable but also improves digestion and promotes healthier eating habits. Likewise, mindful walking involves feeling the ground beneath your feet and noticing the sights and sounds around you. These activities help integrate mindfulness seamlessly into daily life, providing continuous stress relief and emotional support.

While mindfulness meditation has many benefits, it is essential to remember that consistency is key. Regular practice leads to more significant improvements in stress management and overall health. For caregivers and family members, encouraging seniors to adopt a consistent mindfulness routine can make a substantial difference in their loved ones' quality of life. Health professionals can also play a crucial role by recommending mindfulness practices tailored to the individual needs of their senior patients.

To support seniors in building a robust mindfulness practice, creating a dedicated space for meditation can be beneficial. Choose a quiet, comfortable area free from distractions. Use this space solely for mindfulness exercises to establish a strong association between the environment and the practice. Over time, just entering this space can signal to the brain that it's time to relax and focus.

Additionally, seniors should feel encouraged to explore different types of mindfulness practices to find what works best for them. Guided meditation sessions, available online or through mobile apps, provide structure and support, especially for beginners. Group classes can also offer community and motivation, enhancing the overall experience.

Family members and caregivers can further assist by joining in mindfulness activities, fostering a supportive environment where everyone benefits from reduced stress and improved emotional well-being. Sharing these practices can strengthen relationships and create a more harmonious living situation.

Starting a Meditation Practice

Starting a mindfulness meditation practice at home can be an enriching journey, especially for seniors. This guide offers tips and insights to help you begin with ease and confidence.

Begin with just a few minutes each day. It's important to know that you don't need to meditate for hours to reap the benefits of mindfulness. Start small - even five minutes a day can make a difference. This short duration can easily fit into your daily routine without feeling overwhelming. For example, consider pairing your meditation with a daily activity you already do regularly, like having your morning coffee (dwitt@linkwellhealth.com, 2022).

Simple guidance can help you feel more comfortable with the process. There's no one right way to meditate. You can sit on a chair, lie down, or even stand if sitting is uncomfortable. The key is to find a position where you feel supported and at ease. Focus on your breathing. Pay attention to the gentle rise and fall of your chest or the sensation of air flowing through your nose. This focus helps anchor you in the present moment, reducing feelings of anxiety and stress.

Regular practice can create a strong foundation for managing stress effec-tively. Consistency is vital in building any new habit, and meditation is no different. Try to find a specific time of day that works best for you, whether it's early in the morning, in the afternoon, or before bedtime. Setting aside this dedicated time every day will help meditation become a natural part of your routine. Over time, you'll likely notice an improved ability to handle stress and a greater sense of calm and well-being. Establishing a routine is crucial – it signals your mind that it's time to relax and focus. Consider using a timer or a meditation app to ensure you meditate for your intended duration and not worry about watching the clock (dwitt@linkwellhealth.com, 2022).

Incorporate simple activities to integrate mindfulness seamlessly into your everyday life. Mindfulness doesn't have to happen only during seated meditation sessions. Activities such as mindful walking or eating can bring mindfulness into your daily routine. When walking, pay attention to the sensation of your feet touching the ground, the rhythm of your steps, or the sounds around you. This brings a meditative quality to the act of walking, transforming it from a mundane task into a mindful experience.

Mindful eating is another excellent way to practice mindfulness throughout the day. Rather than rushing through meals, take the time to savor each bite. Notice the flavors, textures, and aromas of your food. This not only enhances your enjoyment of eating but also helps promote healthy digestion and awareness of your body's hunger and fullness cues. Eating mindfully can also lead to better food choices, contributing to overall well-being.

An essential aspect of starting a mindfulness meditation practice is creating a conducive environment at home. Find a quiet spot where you won't be disturbed. This could be a corner of your living room, a cozy chair by a window, or even your bedroom. Make this space inviting and free from clutter. Some people find adding soft lighting, candles, or soothing music helps create a serene atmosphere. Having a designated meditation spot can signal your brain that it's time to unwind and relax, making it easier to slip into meditation mode.

Remember, there's no need for special equipment or attire. Wear whatever feels comfortable, and sit or lie down in a way that supports your back and allows you to breathe openly. The goal is to reduce any physical discomforts so you can focus entirely on the meditation practice.

As you grow more comfortable with meditation, you might explore different techniques to see what suits you best. For beginners, a popular method is Box

Breathing: breathe in slowly for four counts, hold your breath for four counts, breathe out slowly for four counts, hold your breath for four counts, then repeat. This technique can help regulate your breathing and create a sense of calm.

Approaching meditation with openness and curiosity is essential. Understand that it's normal for your mind to wander. Don't get frustrated when it happens; gently bring your attention back to your breath or chosen focus point. This practice of returning your attention strengthens your mindfulness skills over time. Be kind and patient with yourself during this learning process. Mindfulness meditation isn't about achieving perfect stillness but about observing your thoughts and feelings with acceptance and without judgment.

For those who prefer guided support, consider using mindfulness meditation apps. Many apps offer beginner-friendly sessions that walk you through different meditation practices. Popular apps include Headspace, Calm, and Ten Percent Happier. These tools can provide structure and variety to your meditation routine, making it easier to stay engaged and motivated.

Deep Breathing Exercises

Deep breathing techniques provide an immediate and effective way to alleviate stress, making them ideal for seniors managing diabetes. Controlled breathing can trigger the body's relaxation response, significantly reducing stress hormones like cortisol. This response is essential for individuals with diabetes as stress can adversely affect blood sugar levels.

One particularly beneficial deep breathing technique is the 4-7-8 method. Originating from the yogic practice of pranayama, this method has been popularized for its simplicity and effectiveness. The 4-7-8 technique involves inhaling through the nose for four counts, holding the breath for seven counts, and exhaling through the mouth for eight counts. Practicing this method regularly can help train the nervous system to shift from a state of stress to one of relaxation more efficiently (Cleveland Clinic, 2022).

Incorporating the 4-7-8 breathing technique into a daily routine is straightforward and can be done almost anywhere. It's especially useful during high-stress moments, such as checking blood sugar levels. Stressful situations can cause a spike in blood glucose, but employing the 4-7-8 method before or after testing can help maintain calmness and stabilize those levels.

Staying hydrated is another critical factor that supports respiratory health and overall well-being. Adequate hydration keeps the mucous membranes in the respiratory tract moist, which is vital for efficient breathing. Seniors often face challenges related to dry mouth and throat, increasing the effort required for breathing. Drinking water throughout the day ensures smoother respiration and, consequently, better stress management. Moreover, dehydration can lead to increased blood sugar levels, making it doubly important for diabetics to stay hydrated.

The benefits of controlled breathing extend beyond immediate stress relief. Regular practice helps in training the body to respond better to stress over time. Engaging in the 4-7-8 technique consistently enables the parasympathetic nervous system, responsible for rest and digestion, to take control more effectively, counterbalancing the fight-or-flight response triggered by the sympathetic nervous system. This balance is crucial for maintaining emotional and physical health.

Guidelines for practicing the 4-7-8 breathing technique are simple enough for anyone to follow. Here's how you can incorporate this method into your daily life:

1. Find a Comfortable Position: Sit up straight if possible. If you're using the technique to fall asleep, lying down works too.
2. Position Your Tongue: Keep your tongue resting against the roof of your mouth, just behind your front teeth.
3. Exhale Completely: Start with a deep exhale through your mouth, making a whooshing sound.
4. Inhale and Count to Four: Breathe in quietly through your nose while mentally counting to four.
5. Hold and Count to Seven: Hold your breath for a count of seven.
6. Exhale and Count to Eight: Breathe out completely through your mouth, making a whoosh sound for a count of eight.

Repeating these steps for four cycles takes only about a minute but can provide profound calming effects almost immediately. With continued practice, this technique becomes a powerful tool for quickly alleviating stress.

Encouraging practices such as deep breathing during high-stress moments can make a significant difference in health outcomes for seniors with diabetes. Monitoring blood sugar levels can be stressful, but employing these techniques can transform a potentially anxiety-inducing activity into a moment of calmness and control. This not only helps in managing stress but also positively impacts blood sugar levels.

Additionally, incorporating other minor adjustments, like staying hydrated, can further enhance the effectiveness of breathing exercises. Drinking adequate water supports respiratory health, making it easier to perform deep breathing exercises. Proper hydration also aids in maintaining balanced blood sugar levels, which is crucial for diabetes management.

Creating a Stress-Free Environment

Environmental factors play a crucial role in managing stress and diabetes. Understanding how our immediate surroundings impact our well-being is essential for seniors and caregivers aiming to create calming, supportive environments.

First, it's important to recognize the impact of clutter and distractions on stress levels. A cluttered space can lead to sensory overload, making it difficult to focus and relax. For seniors managing diabetes, this added stress can exacerbate symptoms and complicate daily routines. To address this, start by evaluating your living spaces. Take note of areas where items tend to accumulate and consider implementing simple organizational systems. By keeping surfaces clear and having designated places for frequently used items, you can reduce mental clutter and create a more serene environment.

Adding calming elements to your home can significantly enhance relaxation. Simple decor changes, such as incorporating plants, artwork, or soft lighting, can create a soothing atmosphere. Indoor plants not only add a touch of nature but also improve air quality, contributing to a sense of well-being. Choose easy-to-care-for plants like snake plants or succulents if upkeep is a concern. Similarly, artwork that evokes positive emotions can serve as a visual reminder to pause and breathe. Soft lighting, achieved through lamps or candles, can replace harsh overhead lights, creating a cozy, inviting space perfect for unwinding.

Reducing exposure to negative news or stressful social interactions is another critical step in managing stress. Constantly consuming negative media can heighten anxiety and create a cycle of worry. Consider setting boundaries for news consumption, such as limiting it to specific times of the day or opting for written articles over continuous television coverage. Additionally, be mindful of social interactions that may be draining or stressful. Surround yourself with supportive, positive people and engage in activities that bring joy and relaxation. By consciously choosing what media to consume and who to spend time with, you can protect your mental health and maintain a more balanced state of mind.

Nature has been shown to significantly lower stress and improve mood. Spending time outdoors or even bringing elements of nature inside can have a profound impact on mental health. Studies suggest that being in green spaces can reduce cortisol levels, the body's primary stress hormone, and promote feelings of calm. If mobility is an issue, consider small changes like opening windows to let in natural light and fresh air, or placing bird feeders near windows for a connection to wildlife. Even viewing scenes of nature, whether through photographs or videos, can trigger similar stress-reducing benefits.

Incorporating these environmental adjustments doesn't require drastic changes. Small steps can lead to meaningful improvements in stress management and overall health. By assessing your space, introducing calming elements, minimizing stress triggers, and embracing nature, you can create a supportive environment that enhances well-being and aids in managing diabetes effectively.

Guidelines:

1. **Assessing Your Space**: Start by evaluating your current environment. Identify areas that feel chaotic or stressful and make a plan to declutter and organize. Small changes, like sorting mail immediately or designating a spot for keys, can make a significant difference.

2. **Incorporating Calming Elements**: Introduce decor that promotes relaxation. Consider adding plants like aloe vera or peace lilies, which are known for their air-purifying qualities. Choose artwork that brings you joy and arrange lighting to create a warm, inviting ambiance.

3. **Limiting Stress Triggers**: Be mindful of your media consumption. Set limits on how often you check the news and curate your social media feeds to emphasize positive content. When interacting with others, prioritize relationships that uplift and support you.

4. **Using Nature**: Make a conscious effort to incorporate nature into your daily life. Spend time outside whenever possible, whether it's a walk in the park or sitting on your porch. If outdoor activities are limited, bring nature indoors with houseplants, natural light, and fresh air.

Final Insights

This chapter has highlighted the power of mindfulness meditation and relaxation techniques to help seniors manage stress effectively, a vital component in diabetes care. By practicing mindfulness and staying in the present moment, seniors can alleviate anxiety and enhance emotional resilience. This approach also aids in recognizing and addressing specific stress triggers, thus promoting a calmer and more balanced lifestyle. With benefits extending from lower blood pressure to improved cognitive function, consistent mindfulness practice becomes an invaluable tool in one's daily routine.

Encouraging seniors to cultivate mindfulness through simple steps like mindful breathing, eating, and walking can make a substantial difference in their overall well-being. Caregivers and family members play a crucial role in supporting these practices, ensuring that seniors have the resources and motivation needed to maintain their routines. Health professionals can further guide by recommending tailored mindfulness exercises. Creating a supportive environment where mindfulness is practiced regularly not only helps in managing stress but also strengthens relationships and enhances the quality of life for everyone involved.

$$5$$

Quality Sleep: The Foundation of Health

Quality sleep is the foundation of health, especially for seniors managing diabetes. Without adequate and restorative sleep, overall well-being can suffer, making it harder to manage blood sugar levels and stay healthy. Sleep affects nearly every aspect of our lives, from mood and cognitive function to physical health and immune response. That's why focusing on enhancing sleep quality is not just a luxury but a necessity for people in this age group who are dealing with the challenges of diabetes management.

This chapter delves into practical and effective strategies to enhance sleep quality through a structured bedtime routine. You'll learn the importance of maintaining consistent sleep and wake times to align your body's natural rhythms. Additionally, we'll discuss relaxing activities like reading and light stretching to help ease you into a state of relaxation before bed. We'll also highlight the significance of reducing screen time and creating a sleep-friendly environment by ensuring your bedroom is dark, cool, and quiet. Together, these habits form a comprehensive approach to improving sleep quality and, by extension, better managing diabetes and overall health.

Creating a Bedtime Routine

Establishing a calming bedtime routine is fundamental to improving sleep quality, especially for seniors managing diabetes. A consistent routine helps signal the body that it is time to wind down and prepare for restful sleep, which is crucial for overall well-being. One of the primary ways to achieve this is by maintaining regular sleep and wake times. Consistency in these habits helps regulate the body's internal clock, also known as the circadian rhythm, making it easier to fall asleep at night and wake up feeling refreshed. For example, if you go to bed and get up at the same time every day, including weekends, your body becomes accustomed to this schedule, allowing you to enjoy a more natural and restorative sleep cycle.

Another effective way to enhance relaxation before bedtime is by incorporating gentle activities such as reading or light stretching. These activities help ease the mind and body into a state of relaxation, making it simpler to transition to sleep. Reading a book provides a mental escape and reduces stress levels, while light stretching can help relieve muscle tension accumulated throughout the day. This gentle exercise promotes physical relaxation without causing overstimulation. For instance, spending 20 minutes reading a favorite novel or doing a series of simple stretches designed to relax muscles can make a significant difference in preparing the body for a good night's sleep.

Reducing screen time before bed is also critical. The blue light emitted from devices like smartphones, tablets, and computers can disrupt the production of melatonin, a hormone that regulates sleep. Melatonin is naturally produced by the body in response to darkness and helps signal that it is time to sleep. However, exposure to blue light can delay melatonin production, making it harder for individuals to fall asleep. Therefore, it's crucial to establish a technology curfew, ideally turning off all screens at least an hour before bedtime. If completely avoiding screens isn't feasible, using blue light filters or switching to audio-based content like white noise or soothing music can be beneficial. Studies show that limiting screen time during the 30 to 60 minutes before bedtime can yield modest benefits in terms of "lights out" time as well as sleep quality and duration (*Does Screen Time before Bed Actually Affect Your Sleep?*, 2023).

To create a sleep-inducing environment, ensure the bedroom is dark, cool, and quiet. A dark room promotes melatonin production, further facilitating the onset of sleep. Using blackout curtains or a sleep mask can be effective ways to block unwanted light. Additionally, maintaining a comfortably cool temperature in the bedroom can improve sleep efficiency. Most people sleep better when the room is slightly cooler, as the body's core temperature naturally drops to initiate sleep. A quiet space is equally important; minimizing noise disruptions can significantly enhance sleep quality. If external noises are unavoidable, consider using earplugs or a white noise machine to create a more peaceful environment conducive to sleep.

Adopting these practices can result in substantial improvements in sleep quality. For example, a senior who sticks to a regular bedtime, engages in relaxing pre-sleep activities, avoids screens before bed, and optimizes their sleeping environment is likely to experience better sleep. This, in turn, supports more effective diabetes management by regulating blood sugar levels and reducing stress. Good sleep hygiene practices, therefore, become an integral part of a holistic approach to health for seniors and those caring for them.

Creating a routine that consistently signals the body it's time to wind down can have profound effects on sleep quality. Regular sleep and wake times align the body's intrinsic rhythms with the external environment, promoting better sleep patterns. Gentle activities like reading or stretching offer physical and mental relaxation, paving the way for a smoother transition into sleep. Reducing screen exposure before bed safeguards against melatonin disruption, ensuring the body's natural sleep cues remain intact. Finally, crafting a dark, cool, and quiet bedroom environment eliminates potential disturbances, fostering a setting where uninterrupted sleep can flourish.

Optimizing Sleep Environment

Enhancing the environment in which you sleep is essential to promoting restorative rest and can greatly improve overall health, particularly for seniors managing diabetes. By making targeted physical changes to your bedroom, you can create a space that encourages deeper, more refreshing sleep. Here are some effective strategies to consider:

Maintaining an optimal sleeping temperature is crucial for restful sleep. A cooler room helps lower your body temperature, supporting various stages of the sleep cycle. The ideal temperature range is usually between 60-67 degrees Fahrenheit. If this feels too cold, adding extra layers to your bedding or opting for warmer pajamas can help. Conversely, during warmer weather, consider removing layers or using lighter bedclothes to maintain a comfortable sleeping environment.

Noise pollution can be a substantial barrier to achieving quality sleep. Loud noises can disrupt sleep patterns and cause frequent awakenings, leading to reduced sleep quality. To mitigate noise issues, employing earplugs, white noise machines, or even soft background music can substantially reduce disturbances. These tools can mask sudden sounds and create a more consistent auditory environment conducive to uninterrupted sleep. For those who find these methods uncomfortable, thick curtains or carpets can also absorb sound and lessen noise levels.

Ensuring your room is dark enough is another important aspect of creating a restful sleep environment. Darkness promotes the production of melatonin, a hormone that regulates sleep-wake cycles. Investing in blackout curtains can effectively block outside light, ensuring your room remains dark throughout the night. If complete darkness feels unsettling, consider using a small, dim nightlight that maintains low light levels without disrupting melatonin production.

Comfort plays a significant role in sleep quality, and investing in high-quality bedding can make a noticeable difference. A supportive mattress and pillows tailored to your specific comfort needs can alleviate pressure points and reduce discomfort. Memory foam mattresses, for example, conform to your body's shape, providing both support and relief for joint pain, which is commonly experienced by seniors. Additionally, pillows that support your neck and align your spine can prevent aches and improve overall sleep posture.

Understanding Sleep Cycles

Understanding the different stages of sleep is crucial for recognizing their significance in overall health and diabetes management. Sleep is categorized into two main types: REM (rapid eye movement) sleep and non-REM (non-rapid eye movement) sleep. These two types are further divided into various stages. Non-REM sleep includes three stages: N1, N2, and N3, with each playing a unique role in the restorative processes of the body.

Stage N1 is the lightest stage of sleep where one can be easily awakened. It's a brief period, typically lasting just a few minutes, serving as the transition from wakefulness to sleep. Stage N2 follows, constituting about 50% of our total sleep time. During N2, heart rate and breathing stabilize, and the body temperature drops, setting the stage for deeper sleep. Stage N3, also known as deep sleep, is essential for physical restoration and immune function. It's during this stage that the body repairs tissues, builds bone and muscle, and strengthens the immune system. On the other hand, REM sleep is characterized by rapid movements of the eyes, more vivid dreams, and heightened brain activity. It plays a significant role in cognitive functions like memory consolidation, learning, and emotional regulation.

Achieving an adequate amount of each sleep stage is vital for maintaining optimal health. For individuals managing diabetes or those at risk, this becomes even more critical. Studies have shown that disrupted sleep architecture—wherein the balance of sleep stages is altered—can adversely impact glucose metabolism. This disruption can lead to reduced insulin sensitivity, subsequently elevating blood sugar levels. Consistently shortchanging oneself on sleep can provoke insulin resistance, a precursor to type 2 diabetes.

To harness the full benefits of sleep, aiming for 7-9 hours of sleep per night is recommended. This duration allows sufficient time for the body to cycle through all the necessary stages of sleep multiple times. Achieving regular sleep duration requires adjusting various lifestyle habits. For seniors, this might mean establishing a consistent bedtime routine, which can signal the body that it's time to wind down and prepare for sleep. Cutting back on caffeine and heavy meals before bedtime and creating a comfortable sleep environment can also play a substantial role in enhancing sleep quality.

A lack of sleep can have immediate and prolonged effects on blood sugar levels. Studies have illustrated that even a single night of inadequate sleep can result in higher blood glucose levels the following day. Over time, this can exacerbate blood sugar control, making diabetes management more challenging. The relationship between sleep and diabetes is bidirectional; poor sleep can worsen diabetes symptoms, while diabetes can lead to sleep disturbances. Symptoms such as frequent urination during the night, nighttime hypoglycemia, and discomfort from neuropathy can further disrupt sleep, creating a vicious cycle.

Given the critical link between sleep and diabetes, implementing effective sleep strategies becomes paramount. One useful approach is monitoring sleep patterns. Using tools such as sleep diaries or wearable sleep trackers can help individuals recognize trends in their sleep behavior. For example, noting the duration and quality of sleep each night helps pinpoint factors that may be affecting sleep, whether it's specific foods, medications, or stressors. Recognizing these patterns makes it easier to make targeted adjustments.

Furthermore, tracking one's sleep can offer valuable data when consulting healthcare professionals. Health providers can use this information to develop personalized recommendations that enhance sleep quality and, consequently, improve diabetes management. Simple interventions such as optimizing medication schedules to prevent nocturnal hypoglycemia or suggesting timely carbohydrate intake can significantly reduce sleep disruptions.

Implementing these practices can substantially improve not only sleep quality but also overall health outcomes. Ensuring that one gets adequate, high-quality sleep supports better blood sugar control, enhances mood, and boosts cognitive function. For caregivers and family members, encouraging loved ones to prioritize sleep can be a powerful way to support their health journey. Reminding them gently about the importance of sleep, helping them establish a bedtime routine, and ensuring a conducive sleep environment are steps that can make a tangible difference.

Addressing Sleep Disruptions

As we age, maintaining a good night's sleep can become increasingly difficult due to various factors that disrupt our rest. Understanding and addressing these issues are vital for overall well-being and effective diabetes management in seniors. This section will explore strategies to identify common sleep disruptions and provide practical solutions to improve sleep quality.

One major factor that affects sleep in seniors is medication. Many older adults take multiple medications for different health conditions, and some of these can interfere with sleep. For instance, certain heart medications, antidepressants, and corticosteroids are known to cause insomnia or restless sleep. It's essential to review all medications with your healthcare provider to determine if any may be contributing to sleep disturbances. Sometimes, adjusting the timing of medication intake or switching to an alternative prescription can make a significant difference.

Pain is another common issue that disrupts sleep among seniors. Conditions such as arthritis, neuropathy, and chronic back pain can make it challenging to find a comfortable sleeping position, leading to frequent awakenings during the night. Using specialized pillows or mattresses designed to alleviate pressure points can help. Additionally, engaging in regular gentle exercises like stretching or yoga can improve flexibility and reduce pain over time, making it easier to sleep through the night.

Anxiety and stress are also prevalent among seniors and can significantly impact sleep quality. Worrying about health, family matters, or financial issues can lead to racing thoughts that keep individuals awake at night. Techniques such as gentle breathing exercises or journaling before bed can help mitigate anxious thoughts. Breathing exercises involve taking slow, deep breaths to calm the mind and body, while journaling allows one to write down worries, thereby releasing them from the mind. These practices create a more relaxed state conducive to falling asleep.

In some cases, it is crucial to seek professional help to address sleep disruptions effectively. If you consistently struggle with sleep despite trying various techniques, it may be time to consult healthcare professionals. A doctor can evaluate whether there are underlying medical conditions, such as sleep apnea or restless leg syndrome, which require specific treatments. Sleep studies conducted by specialists can provide detailed insights into your sleep patterns and identify potential disorders that need targeted interventions. Consulting a mental health professional can also be beneficial if anxiety or depression is significantly impacting your sleep quality. Receiving appropriate treatment for these conditions can improve both mental health and sleep.

Making minor lifestyle adjustments can also support better sleep hygiene. Diet plays a crucial role in sleep quality. Consuming large meals close to bedtime can cause discomfort and indigestion, making it difficult to fall asleep. Opt for lighter meals in the evening, and avoid caffeine and alcohol late in the day, as they can interfere with sleep. Instead, choose calming herbal teas like chamomile, which promote relaxation without the stimulant effects of caffeine.

Physical activity is another key component of improving sleep hygiene. Regular exercise helps regulate the sleep-wake cycle and enhances overall physical health, making it easier to fall and stay asleep. However, it's important to schedule exercise earlier in the day, as vigorous activity close to bedtime can be stimulating and counterproductive to sleep. Aim for activities that suit your fitness level, such as walking, swimming, or tai chi, which provide both physical and mental benefits.

Sleep environment modifications can further enhance sleep quality. Ensure your bedroom is conducive to sleep by maintaining a comfortable temperature, minimizing noise, and keeping the room dark. Consider using earplugs or white noise machines to block out disruptive sounds and blackout curtains to prevent light from entering the room. Investing in a quality mattress and pillows can also contribute to a restful night's sleep, providing the necessary support and comfort to alleviate pressure points and reduce pain.

Cognitive Behavioral Therapy for Insomnia (CBT-I) is another effective method for treating sleep problems. CBT-I focuses on identifying and changing negative thoughts and behaviors that contribute to sleep difficulties. Working with a trained therapist, you can develop healthier sleep habits and coping mechanisms to manage anxiety and stress. Incorporating mindfulness and relaxation techniques into your daily routine can also support better sleep by promoting a calm and peaceful mindset before bedtime.

Maintaining a consistent sleep schedule is paramount for regulating the body's internal clock. Go to bed and wake up at the same time every day, even on weekends, to establish a regular rhythm. Avoid napping in the late afternoon or evening, as this can interfere with nighttime sleep. Developing a soothing pre-sleep routine, such as reading a book, listening to calming music, or taking a warm bath, signals the body that it's time to wind down and prepare for sleep.

For seniors managing diabetes, blood sugar levels can also impact sleep quality. High or low blood sugar levels can cause discomfort and frequent awakenings. Monitor your blood sugar levels regularly and follow your healthcare provider's recommendations to keep them within target ranges. Eating a balanced diet and staying hydrated throughout the day can help stabilize blood sugar levels, reducing nocturnal disturbances.

Final Thoughts

Improving sleep quality is a cornerstone of overall well-being and effective diabetes management, and this chapter has highlighted several strategies to achieve this. By establishing a calming bedtime routine through consistent sleep and wake times, engaging in relaxing activities before bed, reducing screen time, and optimizing the sleep environment, seniors can experience significant enhancements in their sleep patterns. These practices not only aid in falling asleep more easily but also contribute to more restorative and uninterrupted sleep, which is vital for regulating blood sugar levels and reducing stress.

Ultimately, adopting these sleep-promoting habits can lead to tangible benefits for both physical and mental health. A good night's sleep helps manage diabetes more effectively by maintaining stable blood glucose levels and improving mood and cognitive function. For caregivers, supporting loved ones in creating and maintaining these routines is a powerful way to enhance their quality of life. Prioritizing sleep hygiene is a simple yet profound step toward achieving better health outcomes, making it an invaluable addition to any diabetes management plan.

6

Hydration Habits: The Key Role of Water

Staying well-hydrated is one of the simplest yet most powerful habits for effective diabetes management. Proper hydration plays a critical role in our bodies by aiding in the regulation of blood sugar levels, supporting kidney function, and maintaining overall health. Drinking enough water can help stabilize blood viscosity, enabling vital organs to perform their functions more efficiently. This chapter underscores how adequate water intake can make a significant difference in managing diabetes and improving general well-being.

Throughout this chapter, you will discover the numerous benefits linked to staying hydrated, from enhancing energy levels to supporting physical activity. We'll explore how proper hydration aids digestion, prevents fatigue, and even has cognitive advantages that are essential for seniors. Additionally, you'll learn tips on increasing your daily water consumption and recognizing signs of dehydration. Whether you are a senior managing diabetes, a caregiver, or a healthcare professional, the insights provided here will guide you towards better hydration habits, ultimately leading to improved health outcomes.

Benefits of Proper Hydration

The relationship between hydration and diabetes management is crucial, with numerous benefits linked to proper hydration. Staying well-hydrated helps to regulate blood viscosity, which in turn aids the kidneys in filtering blood more effectively. This process is essential for keeping blood sugar levels stable, as the kidneys play a critical role in excreting excess glucose through urine. When you drink enough water, you support this natural filtering mechanism, thereby promoting better blood sugar control.

Hydration also has a direct impact on energy levels. Adequate water intake prevents fatigue, making it easier to engage in physical activities that are beneficial for managing diabetes. When your body is dehydrated, it can lead to feelings of lethargy and tiredness, which can hinder your ability to stay active. Physical activity is a key component in diabetes management because it helps reduce blood sugar levels by increasing insulin sensitivity. Therefore, by staying hydrated, you not only feel more energetic but also enhance your ability to maintain an active lifestyle, which is vital for managing diabetes effectively.

In addition to supporting physical activity, proper hydration is essential for kidney function. Kidneys are responsible for removing waste products and excess fluids from the body, and they require sufficient water intake to operate efficiently. Dehydration can put undue stress on the kidneys, potentially leading to complications such as kidney stones or even chronic kidney disease, both of which are common among people with diabetes (Nakamura et al., 2020). By ensuring adequate water intake, you help protect your kidneys from these complications, thereby improving your overall health and making diabetes management more effective.

Another significant benefit of staying hydrated is its positive effect on digestion. Proper hydration aids in the digestive process by helping break down food, preventing constipation, and facilitating nutrient absorption. When your body is well-hydrated, it can more efficiently absorb essential nutrients from the food you eat, which is particularly important for individuals with diabetes who need to carefully manage their diet. Constipation can be a common issue among those with diabetes due to fluctuations in blood sugar levels and medication side effects. Drinking enough water can alleviate this problem by keeping the digestive system functioning smoothly.

The advantages of maintaining proper hydration extend beyond just physical health; there are cognitive benefits as well. Mild dehydration has been shown to affect mood and cognitive functions, leading to issues like irritability and difficulty concentrating. For seniors managing diabetes, these cognitive effects can add an extra layer of challenge. Staying adequately hydrated can improve mental clarity, making it easier to follow diabetes management plans and make informed decisions about diet and exercise.

Proper hydration also supports the body's ability to manage stress and metabolic functions. Water plays a vital role in virtually every physiological process, including the regulation of hormones that help control stress and metabolism. Dehydration can disrupt these processes, making it harder to manage stress and maintain stable metabolic functions. For those with diabetes, where stress and metabolic imbalance can directly impact blood sugar levels, staying hydrated is an essential part of overall health management.

Given these benefits, it's clear that hydration should be a priority for anyone managing diabetes. Integrating consistent water intake into daily routines can be a simple yet powerful tool for improving health outcomes. Health professionals working with seniors should emphasize the importance of hydration as part of a comprehensive diabetes management plan. Caregivers and family members can support their loved ones by encouraging regular water consumption and providing reminders.

While drinking water may seem like a straightforward habit, it's one that carries profound implications for health, especially for those managing diabetes. The simple act of reaching for a glass of water can support blood sugar regulation, enhance energy levels, protect kidney function, aid digestion, and even improve cognitive function. By understanding and prioritizing hydration, individuals can take a significant step towards better diabetes management and overall well-being.

Tips for Increasing Water Intake

Boosting water consumption throughout the day is crucial for seniors, particularly those managing diabetes. Here are practical strategies to help increase hydration, ensuring health benefits like stable blood sugar levels and overall well-being.

Setting Reminders

One of the simplest yet highly effective strategies is setting reminders for hydration. For seniors, technology can be a valuable ally in this regard. Using phone alarms or reminder apps can serve as gentle nudges throughout the day to drink water. If smartphones aren't convenient, sticky notes placed strategically around the home—in areas like the kitchen, bathroom, and living room—can also serve as great visual cues. These constant reminders can make it easier to incorporate regular drinking habits into daily routines.

Infusing Water with Flavors

Drinking plain water can sometimes be monotonous, making it challenging to meet daily hydration goals. However, adding natural flavors can significantly enhance its appeal. Infusing water with fruits such as lemon, lime, strawberries, or herbs like mint and basil can transform a bland beverage into a refreshing treat. Not only does this make drinking more enjoyable, but it also adds a hint of vitamins and antioxidants from the added fruits and herbs. This method can be a delightful solution for seniors who find plain water unappealing.

Using Refillable Water Bottles

A practical tip to ensure consistent hydration is using a refillable water bottle. Carrying a water bottle encourages regular sipping throughout the day and helps track daily intake. Seniors can choose a bottle with measurement markers to monitor how much they have consumed by specific times of the day, ensuring they meet their hydration goals. Moreover, keeping the bottle within arm's reach, whether at home or on the go, eliminates the barriers to drinking water, making it a seamless part of their routine.

Integrating Water Intake with Meals

Incorporating water consumption into mealtimes is another effective strategy. Drinking a glass of water before, during, and after meals not only aids digestion but also ensures that hydration is consistent throughout the day. This habit can be effortlessly integrated into existing routines, making it less likely to be forgotten. Additionally, having water readily available during meals can help reduce the temptation to opt for sugary or caffeinated drinks, which can negatively impact blood sugar levels.

Practical Examples and Tips

Beyond these core strategies, there are other creative ways to boost water intake. For instance, tying hydration to routine activities can be very effective.

Seniors might get into the habit of drinking a glass of water every time they brush their teeth, finish a chapter of a book, or complete a household chore. This method ensures that they are regularly reminded to hydrate without needing extra external prompts.

Also, engaging in social activities that promote drinking water can be beneficial. For example, participating in group activities where everyone is encouraged to bring their water bottles can turn hydration into a shared goal, providing both a community support system and a sense of accountability.

Another practical tip for caregivers is to make water accessible. Placing pitchers of infused water in common areas of the house can serve as an inviting reminder. Similarly, providing seniors with lightweight, easy-to-hold cups can remove physical barriers and make it easier for them to drink independently.

Combining Strategies for Best Results

Combining these strategies can yield even better results. For instance, a senior could set a phone alarm to remind them to drink water and have a refillable bottle with them at all times. They might also infuse their water with fruits and aim to drink a certain amount with each meal. This multi-faceted approach helps reinforce the habit from multiple angles, making it more likely to stick.

Moreover, involving family members or caregivers in these efforts can enhance success. Family members can help by gently reminding seniors to drink water or by sharing in the activity themselves, making it a collective effort. Caregivers can assist by ensuring that water is always within reach and by encouraging hydration during caregiving tasks, like meal preparation or medication administration.

Addressing Common Challenges

While these strategies are simple, some challenges might still arise. Forgetfulness can be a significant barrier, especially for those dealing with cognitive impairments. In such cases, establishing a structured routine around hydration can be highly beneficial. Consistency in timing, such as always drinking water after waking up, can create a habitual pattern that becomes second nature over time.

Physical limitations can also pose challenges. Seniors with arthritis or mobility issues might find it difficult to handle heavy pitchers or constantly move to get water. Adaptive tools like lightweight, ergonomic bottles or cups with easy-grip handles can alleviate these issues, allowing for greater independence and ease.

Finally, it's important to celebrate small victories in this journey toward better hydration. Recognizing improvements—whether it's an increase in daily water intake or fewer moments of feeling dehydrated—can provide motivation and reinforce the importance of staying hydrated.

Conclusion

Boosting daily water consumption is essential for seniors, especially those managing diabetes. Practical strategies like setting reminders, infusing water with flavors, using refillable bottles, and integrating water intake with meals can significantly enhance hydration habits. By making these practices a part of their daily routine, seniors can enjoy the myriad health benefits that come with proper hydration, leading to a more active, healthy, and fulfilling life.

Recognizing Signs of Dehydration

Recognizing the early indicators of dehydration is crucial, particularly for seniors managing diabetes. Dehydration can have significant impacts on blood sugar levels and overall health, making it essential to stay vigilant about hydration.

One of the most common and immediate symptoms of dehydration is a dry mouth. This often uncomfortable feeling is your body's way of signaling that it needs more fluids. When you experience a dry or sticky mouth, it's important to drink water promptly. If ignored, this dryness can progress into more severe symptoms and negatively affect your health, particularly if you're managing diabetes.

Fatigue is another prevalent indicator of dehydration. Feeling unusually tired or lethargic can be a sign that your body is not getting enough water. Water is essential for maintaining energy levels, and insufficient hydration can lead to feelings of sluggishness and low energy. For seniors who may already be dealing with fatigue due to other health conditions, recognizing this as a potential symptom of dehydration can prompt timely action.

Dizziness is also a key symptom to watch for. Experiencing dizziness, especially when standing up too quickly, can indicate that your body is dehydrated. This occurs because dehydration reduces blood volume, which in turn can lower blood pressure and cause lightheadedness. If you notice that you frequently feel dizzy upon standing, it's a good idea to increase your water intake to see if the symptoms improve.

Monitoring urine color is a simple yet effective method to gauge hydration levels. Clear to light yellow urine generally indicates proper hydration. Darker urine can be a sign that you need to drink more water. This visual check is an easy and quick way to keep track of your hydration status throughout the day. If you notice consistently dark urine, make it a habit to drink more water regularly.

Postural changes, particularly dizziness when moving from a lying or sitting position to standing, can be a significant sign of dehydration. This type of dizziness happens because blood pressure drops when you stand up quickly, and if your body is lacking adequate fluids, it struggles to adjust. Paying attention to these postural shifts and addressing them by drinking water can help prevent more serious complications.

Another quick check involves examining the mouth and skin for dryness. Dry lips or a sticky feeling in the mouth are clear signs that you might be dehydrated. Additionally, skin that feels less elastic or appears cracked and dry can also indicate fluid loss. These checks are easy to perform and can serve as early warning signs to increase water consumption.

Dehydration doesn't always present immediate or obvious symptoms, so staying proactive is vital. Seniors, in particular, should pay close attention to their bodies and any signs of dehydration, as they are at higher risk due to factors like decreased kidney function and a natural decline in the sense of thirst with age. Caregivers can play an essential role here, reminding their loved ones to drink water regularly and helping monitor for these signs.

Setting up a routine can also help manage hydration effectively. Drinking a glass of water first thing in the morning sets a positive tone for the day. Incorporating water breaks into daily activities, such as drinking water with meals and snacks, ensures consistent hydration. For seniors, who might forget to hydrate, setting reminders or using a refillable water bottle can make keeping track more manageable.

Including hydrating foods in your diet is another approach to maintaining good hydration levels. Foods high in water content, like cucumbers, watermelon, and oranges, provide additional fluids while also offering nutritional benefits. Soups and broths can also contribute to daily fluid intake, particularly in cooler weather when the desire to drink cold water might decrease.

Engaging in regular physical assessments can further aid in monitoring hydration. Simple actions like pinching the skin on the back of your hand to see how quickly it returns to normal can give insight into your hydration status. Slow return can be a sign of dehydration. Similarly, ensuring that you urinate frequently and that the urine is light in color can provide reassurance that you are well-hydrated.

For health professionals working with seniors, it's beneficial to emphasize the importance of hydration in managing diabetes. Providing clear, straightforward advice on how to recognize and address dehydration can empower patients and caregivers alike. Simple educational materials and routines can make a significant difference in promoting better hydration habits.

Avoiding Sugary Drinks

Sugary drinks have become a staple in many diets worldwide, but for seniors managing diabetes, minimizing their consumption in favor of water and healthier alternatives is especially crucial. These sugary beverages, which include sodas, fruit juices, and sweetened teas, can cause significant health issues, particularly concerning blood sugar levels.

Understanding the health risks associated with sugary drink consumption is paramount. These drinks often lead to spikes in blood sugar levels due to their high glycemic index. When consumed, they quickly raise glucose in the bloodstream, prompting a swift insulin response. This can create a cycle of sharp blood sugar increases followed by rapid drops, making blood sugar management challenging for those with diabetes. In addition to affecting blood sugar control, sugary beverages contribute significantly to caloric intake without providing nutritional value, leading to weight gain and obesity, both risk factors for worsening diabetes outcomes. According to research, sugary drinks are among the chief contributors to the obesity and diabetes epidemics in the United States (Sugary Drinks, 2013). Reducing or eliminating these drinks from one's diet can stabilize blood sugar levels and support overall metabolic health.

Encouraging water as the primary beverage choice simplifies healthier decision-making for seniors. Water is calorie-free, helps maintain hydration without impacting blood sugar, and supports various bodily functions. Making water the default beverage during meals and throughout the day can significantly reduce the intake of unnecessary sugars and calories. For those accustomed to the sweetness of sugary drinks, transitioning to water might require an adjustment period. However, the benefits it offers in terms of diabetes management make it a worthwhile shift. It is essential to foster a habit of reaching for water instead of sugary alternatives to maintain consistent hydration and stable blood sugar levels.

Another critical aspect is identifying hidden sugars in drinks by reading labels. Many beverages marketed as healthy, such as fruit juices and sports drinks, contain significant amounts of added sugars that can sabotage diabetes control efforts. Nutritional labels reveal the total amount of sugar per serving, offering insight into how much sugar is being consumed. Seniors and their caregivers can make informed decisions by scrutinizing these labels and opting for drinks with little to no added sugars. This practice not only prevents unwanted blood sugar spikes but also promotes awareness of overall sugar intake. It is essential to recognize that even drinks labeled as "natural" or "organic" can still contain high sugar levels.

Offering healthier alternatives like herbal teas and flavored seltzers can help satisfy cravings without the negative effects of sugary drinks. Herbal teas, available in various flavors, can be enjoyed hot or cold and typically do not contain any sugars or calories. They can be a refreshing change and offer additional health benefits depending on the ingredients. Flavored seltzers provide the pleasant fizz of soda without the added sugars, making them an excellent substitute for those who enjoy carbonated beverages. Infusing water with fruits, vegetables, or herbs can also be a delightful way to enhance its flavor naturally. Adding slices of lemon, cucumber, or mint to water can make it more appealing and encourage increased water consumption.

Cutting back on sugary drinks begins with understanding and recognizing their impact on health. It requires commitment and a strategic approach to replace these beverages with healthier options. Transitioning to water and other low-sugar drinks may take time, but the positive effects on blood sugar control and overall health are substantial. For seniors and caregivers, making these dietary changes can pave the way for better diabetes management and improved quality of life.

In addition to personal efforts, it is beneficial to look at broader actions that can support these individual choices. Beverage manufacturers can play a pivotal role by creating and marketing drinks with lower sugar content. Encouragingly, there is a growing trend among companies to offer products with reduced sugars, catering to health-conscious consumers. Choosing these products when available can reinforce healthier drinking habits.

Families and caregivers should support seniors by ensuring that the home environment emphasizes healthy beverage choices. Stocking the fridge with water, herbal teas, and natural seltzers while avoiding sugary drinks can prevent temptation and make healthier options readily available. Schools and workplaces that cater to seniors should also prioritize offering a range of healthy beverages and provide easy access to fresh, clean water.

Health professionals working with seniors should consistently advocate for reducing sugary drink consumption. Providing clear, simple advice about the benefits of water and healthier alternatives can empower patients to make better choices. By emphasizing practical strategies, such as reading labels and selecting beneficial substitutes, healthcare providers can guide their patients towards sustainable dietary improvements.

Concluding Thoughts

Staying well-hydrated is fundamental for effective diabetes management, as it significantly impacts blood sugar levels and overall health. Proper hydration aids in regulating blood viscosity, supporting kidney function, and facilitating the removal of excess glucose through urine. These processes help maintain stable blood sugar levels, which is crucial for managing diabetes. Additionally, adequate water intake prevents fatigue and promotes physical activity by increasing energy levels and insulin sensitivity. By prioritizing hydration, you enhance your ability to stay active, thus contributing positively to blood sugar control and overall health.

Moreover, the benefits of proper hydration extend beyond physical health and include cognitive and digestive improvements. Staying hydrated can alleviate constipation, facilitate nutrient absorption, and improve mental clarity. For seniors managing diabetes, these benefits are particularly significant, as they support both physical and mental well-being, making it easier to follow diabetes management plans. Encouraging regular water consumption and integrating it into daily routines can greatly enhance health outcomes. Understanding the importance of hydration and making it a priority can empower individuals, caregivers, and health professionals to contribute positively towards better diabetes management and a healthier lifestyle.

7

Building Support Systems: Social Connections Matter

Building a support system is a vital part of staying motivated and managing diabetes effectively. Social connections can be more than just pleasant interactions; they can form the backbone of your health journey. Friends and family provide emotional support and practical help, offering a sense of community that empowers individuals facing challenges. By fostering these relationships, you create an environment where you're not alone in your efforts, making it easier to stick with healthy habits and manage the complexities of diabetes.

This chapter delves into various strategies to strengthen your social connections for better diabetes management. It explores the benefits of open communication with family, engaging in shared activities, and creating a supportive home environment. You'll also learn about the advantages of joining support groups and finding an accountability partner. By understanding how to build and maintain a strong support network, you'll be better equipped to navigate the ups and downs of living with diabetes. This chapter aims to provide practical tips and insights that will help you leverage your social connections to enhance your health and well-being.

Connecting with Family and Friends

Maintaining strong relationships with family and friends plays a crucial role in managing diabetes by providing both emotional support and practical assistance. One of the primary ways to strengthen these bonds is through open communication. Discussing health goals and challenges with family members can create an environment of understanding and encouragement. When seniors openly share their struggles and achievements, it allows their loved ones to offer meaningful support, whether it's through listening, providing advice, or simply being there during difficult times.

Open communication also involves setting clear expectations and sharing knowledge about diabetes management with family members. By educating those around you about the condition, its implications, and the necessary lifestyle changes, you can foster a supportive network. This shared understanding helps reduce misunderstandings and can lead to more cooperative efforts in daily routines that are beneficial for managing diabetes.

Engaging in shared activities is another significant aspect of nurturing social connections. Participating in healthy activities together, such as walking, cooking nutritious meals, or attending fitness classes, can reinforce good habits and make diabetes management less burdensome. These joint activities not only promote physical health but also provide opportunities for bonding and enjoying quality time together. For instance, planning a weekly family hike or a group cooking session can be both fun and beneficial for everyone involved.

In addition to shared activities, regularly checking in with loved ones can make a significant difference in managing diabetes. Regular check-ins, whether through phone calls, visits, or video chats, allow family members and friends to stay informed about your well-being and progress. It also provides a platform for expressing concerns and receiving timely support. These consistent interactions help build a routine of accountability and assurance that someone is always looking out for you.

Creating a supportive environment at home is essential for facilitating effective diabetes management. Family members can play a key role in establishing a home environment conducive to health by making simple yet impactful changes. For example, they can help ensure the availability of healthy foods, assist with meal planning, and encourage regular exercise. A supportive home environment can significantly ease the daily tasks associated with diabetes management and make healthy choices more accessible.

Moreover, family members can assist with practical aspects of diabetes care, such as driving patients to appointments, helping with medication management, or even learning how to monitor blood glucose levels. The involvement of family in these practical tasks not only lightens the load on the individual but also demonstrates a commitment to their health journey, which can be incredibly motivating.

However, it's important to recognize that while family support can be immensely beneficial, it is not without its challenges. Conflicts may arise from differing opinions on how best to manage the condition, and the stress of caregiving can sometimes lead to frustration. Navigating these dynamics requires patience, empathy, and ongoing communication. Families should strive to approach diabetes management as a team effort, respecting each other's perspectives and working towards common goals.

Educating family members about diabetes and its management can alleviate some of these challenges. When family members understand why certain lifestyle changes are necessary, they are better equipped to support those changes. For instance, explaining the importance of a balanced diet and regular exercise can help family members become more active participants in maintaining a healthy household. Resources such as educational workshops, reading materials, or consultations with healthcare professionals can be beneficial in this regard.

Additionally, family-based interventions have been shown to enhance diabetes outcomes. Research indicates that involving family in diabetes education and self-management plans leads to improved adherence to treatment protocols and healthier lifestyle choices (Baig et al., 2016). By empowering families with the right knowledge and skills, they can effectively contribute to better health outcomes for their loved ones living with diabetes.

Joining Support Groups

Joining a diabetes support group can be a game-changer for seniors managing this chronic condition. The shared experiences within these groups can deeply validate your journey, making you feel less isolated in facing diabetes's unique challenges. You hear stories and coping strategies that resonate with your own experiences, underscoring the fact that you are not alone in this fight. This mutual understanding fosters a sense of belonging and normalizes the immense effort required to manage diabetes effectively.

These support groups are also treasure troves of resources. They often provide access to educational materials that may otherwise be hard to find or understand. For instance, members might share diet plans, exercise routines, or advice on medication management, tailored specifically for people with diabetes. Knowing what foods can help stabilize blood sugar levels or learning about new medications from peers who have tried them can be incredibly empowering. This information exchange helps you stay informed and equipped with the latest strategies for managing your condition.

Furthermore, the structure of regular group meetings instills a sense of accountability among participants. When you know others are following up on their health goals and sharing their progress, it creates a subtle pressure to stay committed to your own plans. This collective motivation can significantly improve adherence to treatment regimens, dietary guidelines, and exercise routines. It's much easier to stick to lifestyle changes when you see others successfully navigating similar paths.

Another significant benefit is the social connection formed within these groups. Managing diabetes can sometimes feel like an isolating endeavor, especially if your social circle isn't dealing with the same issues. Being part of a support group means building friendships with people who genuinely understand your struggles. These relationships add a crucial social element to your journey, transforming solo efforts into shared endeavors. As a result, managing diabetes becomes less daunting and more of a communal activity, filled with mutual encouragement and support.

Guidelines for Participation:

1. Find a Local Group: Start by looking for diabetes support groups at local community centers, hospitals, or online forums tailored to seniors.
2. Attend Regularly: Make it a habit to attend meetings consistently to maximize the benefits of shared knowledge and accountability.

3. Engage Actively: Share your experiences and listen to others. Active participation enriches the group dynamic and enhances the learning process.

4. Utilize Offered Resources: Take advantage of any educational materials, workshops, or seminars provided by the group to stay informed and proactive in your diabetes management.

Finding an Accountability Partner

Having a dedicated person to help keep one motivated and on track can significantly impact one's health journey. This section explores how seniors managing diabetes can benefit from having an accountability partner, offering practical guidelines for selecting the right partner, establishing regular check-ins, providing encouragement through challenges, and sharing valuable resources.

Selecting the Right Partner

Choosing the right accountability partner is crucial for success. When selecting someone, it's important to pick a person who understands your health goals and shares a similar level of commitment. This could be a family member, friend, or even a neighbor who has expressed interest in health and wellness. Ideally, this person should have a clear understanding of what it means to manage diabetes, including the lifestyle changes that come with it. Look for someone who is empathetic, reliable, and trustworthy, as these qualities are essential for building a supportive relationship.

For example, you might choose a friend who also has health goals, ensuring mutual understanding and shared experiences. Open communication about both parties' expectations, preferred methods of accountability, and how often to check in will set the foundation for a successful partnership. Psychologist Suzy Reading notes that there are typically two types of accountability partners: mentors who share their wisdom and peers working towards common goals. Choosing the appropriate type for your needs is an essential step.

Regular Check-Ins

Scheduled check-ins play a significant role in maintaining commitment and consistency. Regular intervals for check-ins, whether daily, weekly, or bi-weekly, help ensure that both parties stay motivated and on course. Scheduling specific times for check-ins can foster a sense of responsibility and provide structure to your health management routine. This can include phone calls, video chats, or even meet-ups if circumstances allow.

A study has shown that people are 65% more likely to achieve their goals if they commit to them with someone else, and this likelihood increases to 95% with specific check-ins (Chaudhuri, 2023). These check-ins offer an opportunity to discuss progress, address any challenges, and adjust plans as necessary. Setting a consistent schedule helps create a routine that becomes a natural part of your lifestyle, making it easier to achieve long-term goals.

Encouragement and Challenges

An accountability partner can provide essential encouragement during tough times and present challenges to propel progress. Managing diabetes can sometimes feel overwhelming, especially when dealing with dietary restrictions, medication schedules, or physical activity requirements. Having someone to cheer you on, celebrate small victories, and encourage you when you're feeling discouraged can make a significant difference.

Encouragement goes beyond simple motivational talks; it includes understanding when to push and when to offer empathy. For instance, if you're struggling to stick to an exercise regimen, your partner might suggest trying a new activity together, like walking in a park or attending a fitness class designed for seniors. They can also help by setting up mini-challenges such as cooking a healthy meal together or trying a new recipe that fits dietary restrictions. These activities not only support health goals but also strengthen the bond between partners.

Resource Sharing

Sharing valuable information and resources is another key benefit of having an accountability partner. Managing diabetes involves staying informed about best practices, new treatments, dietary tips, and exercise routines. An accountability partner can help curate and share relevant articles, videos, and other educational materials. This mutual exchange of knowledge ensures that both partners remain well-informed and can make educated decisions about their health.

Resource sharing can take many forms, from forwarding newsletters from trusted medical sources to discussing the latest advice from healthcare providers. It could also involve attending health seminars or webinars together, where both can learn and ask questions. By pooling resources and knowledge, you and your partner can stay ahead of new developments in diabetes care and implement effective strategies to manage the condition better.

Participating in Community Activities

Engaging in local activities can be a powerful way for seniors to enhance their social connections and promote healthy lifestyle choices. One effective approach is finding local groups that cater to health-oriented activities. Community centers often feature a variety of programs designed specifically for seniors, such as walking clubs, fitness classes, and yoga sessions. These groups not only provide opportunities for physical activity but also foster a sense of community and belonging. Joining these programs can be a fun and engaging way to stay active while making new friends. Additionally, local libraries or senior centers may offer book clubs and discussion groups where participants can share experiences and learn from one another.

For those looking to make a difference while enhancing their social connections, volunteering at local charities or organizations can be incredibly fulfilling. Whether it's helping out at a food bank, assisting with community events, or offering skills at local education centers, volunteering provides a sense of purpose and accomplishment. It allows seniors to connect with like-minded individuals, build meaningful relationships, and contribute positively to their communities. This involvement not only enriches the lives of others but also adds structure and routine to daily life, which can be beneficial for mental health.

Participating in community events is another excellent way to enrich social life. Local festivals, fairs, and cultural events provide ample opportunities to meet new people and engage with the community. Attending these events regularly helps seniors feel more connected to their environment and reduces feelings of isolation. Moreover, such events often feature activities that promote physical movement, laughter, and joy, all of which are crucial for maintaining a healthy lifestyle. Seniors can also consider joining hobby-based clubs, like gardening groups or art classes, which align with their interests and allow them to pursue passions while interacting with others.

Many communities offer workshops on healthy living, which can be instrumental in providing both knowledge and motivation for adopting healthier habits. These workshops might cover topics such as nutrition, exercise regimes, stress management, and diabetes care. Attending these workshops not only equips seniors with valuable information but also introduces them to peers who share similar health goals. These educational settings encourage discussions and exchanges of tips and strategies, fostering a supportive environment for everyone involved. It's worth exploring what your local health department or hospitals have to offer, as they frequently organize educational seminars and health screenings tailored to seniors.

Closing Remarks

Connecting with family, friends, and community members is essential for seniors managing diabetes. By fostering strong relationships through open communication and shared activities, seniors can create a supportive environment that promotes healthy habits and makes the management of diabetes less daunting. Whether it's discussing health goals with loved ones or participating in local groups and events, these social connections provide emotional and practical support, making it easier to stay motivated and on track.

Joining diabetes support groups and finding accountability partners offer additional layers of encouragement and resources. These connections can validate your experiences, keep you informed about the latest management strategies, and hold you accountable for your health goals. Engaging in these social structures transforms diabetes management from a solitary task into a communal effort, helping to ensure a more successful and fulfilling health journey.

8

Tracking Progress: Tools and Techniques

racking progress is a vital part of managing diabetes effectively. This chapter explores the powerful role that continuous monitoring plays in enhancing health outcomes for seniors. By keeping track of daily habits, individuals can gain valuable insights into how their actions directly affect blood sugar levels and overall well-being. Awareness fostered through diligent tracking encourages more mindful decisions and empowers seniors to take control of their health journey.

In this chapter, we'll delve into various techniques and tools that make tracking habits more manageable and effective. You'll learn about methods to log daily activities, the benefits of using modern technology like Continuous Glucose Monitoring (CGM) systems, and the psychological boosts from visualizing progress. Additionally, we will discuss how family support and professional guidance can enhance the effectiveness of tracking efforts, making it easier to maintain positive habits over time.

The Importance of Tracking Habits

Tracking progress can profoundly impact the management of diabetes, particularly for seniors. Engaging with tracking tools empowers them to take control of their health by enhancing accountability and motivation. By understanding the significance of each habit and its effect on blood sugar levels, seniors can make informed decisions about their health, fostering a proactive approach to daily management.

Engaging with tracking encourages a deeper understanding of daily habits and their impacts on blood sugar levels. For instance, when a senior monitors their carbohydrate intake, exercise routines, and medication adherence, they begin to see patterns that influence their glucose levels. This awareness allows them to recognize which foods spike their blood sugar or how physical activity helps stabilize it. Such knowledge is vital because it encourages more mindful decisions, ensuring that choices support rather than hinder diabetes management. A senior who notices a consistent rise in blood sugar after consuming certain foods might opt for healthier alternatives, reducing fluctuations and fostering better glycemic control.

Regularly tracking habits fosters a sense of responsibility towards one's health. For many seniors, the act of writing down or logging their daily activities creates a routine that reinforces commitment to their health goals. This sense of duty transcends mere record-keeping; it becomes a personal mission to stay healthy. As they observe their progress over time, seniors feel a stronger obligation to maintain or even improve their health metrics. Furthermore, sharing these logs with healthcare providers or caregivers can provide additional layers of accountability, making seniors more likely to stick to their prescribed plans. For example, a senior who tracks their daily walks and sees improvement in their endurance will likely be motivated to continue exercising, knowing it's contributing positively to their overall wellbeing.

Keeping track provides visible proof of progress, encouraging continued effort. Visual representations of data, like graphs or charts showing blood sugar trends, can be highly motivating. Seeing tangible evidence of improvement or stability can bolster a senior's confidence in their ability to manage diabetes effectively. It also provides reassurance that their efforts are paying off, which is crucial for maintaining long-term commitment. For instance, a senior who consistently records their blood sugar levels and observes gradual lowering of their average readings will feel rewarded for their diligence. This positive reinforcement is essential for sustaining good habits, as it provides both emotional and practical validation of their efforts.

Using tracking data to make informed decisions about necessary adjustments and changes is another critical benefit. When seniors systematically log their health information, they create a valuable resource that can guide future actions. This data-driven approach enables them to identify what works best for their unique circumstances. For instance, if a senior notes that their blood sugar spikes after a specific medication dose, they can discuss this with their healthcare provider to adjust their treatment plan accordingly. Similarly, if a senior realizes that mid-morning snacks help prevent afternoon hypoglycemia, they can incorporate this habit into their daily routine, thereby optimizing their diabetes management strategy.

Moreover, advancements in technology have made tracking more accessible and efficient. Continuous Glucose Monitoring (CGM) systems provide real-time data on glucose levels, allowing for immediate adjustments in insulin dosages and other interventions (Sugandh et al., 2023). These devices eliminate the guesswork and provide accurate, timely feedback, making it easier for seniors to manage their diabetes pro-actively. The integration of CGMs with smartphones and other digital platforms also means that seniors can receive alerts and recommendations, enhancing their ability to respond swiftly to any changes in their condition.

Educational reinforcement through technological devices, such as mobile applications, has also been highlighted as an enabler of diabetes self-management (Adu et al., 2019). These tools offer not only convenience but also comprehensive education, guiding seniors through various aspects of diabetes management. Apps can remind users to check their blood sugar, take medications, and log meals, providing structured support that mitigates the complexities of managing diabetes. This continuous educational interaction ensures that seniors are well-informed and equipped to handle their condition effectively.

Another aspect worth noting is the psychological benefit of tracking. Diabetes management can be overwhelming, especially for seniors who might already be dealing with multiple health issues. Regular tracking simplifies this process by breaking down the task into manageable steps. Each logged entry serves as a small victory, reducing the mental burden and making the overall goal seem more attainable. For example, a senior who tracks their dietary intake might find it easier to follow nutritional guidelines, as the act of recording keeps them mindful of their choices without feeling too restrictive.

Support from caregivers and family members can further enhance the effectiveness of tracking. When caregivers assist with monitoring and interpreting data, it not only eases the senior's workload but also fosters a collaborative environment. Family members can encourage and celebrate milestones, creating a supportive atmosphere that motivates seniors to stay on track. For instance, a caregiver helping a senior review their weekly progress can offer praise for improvements and gently suggest strategies for areas needing attention, reinforcing positive behaviors and addressing challenges constructively.

Using Journals and Diaries

In the journey of managing diabetes, effective journaling can play an instrumental role in tracking daily behaviors and moods. This practice not only facilitates better health management but also enhances overall well-being. Let's delve into the techniques that make journaling a powerful tool for diabetes management.

Daily Log: Highlighting Connections

Creating a simple daily log can be remarkably beneficial. Recording food intake, exercise, and feelings each day helps illuminate patterns and connections between habits and health. By noting what you eat, your physical activities, and how you feel throughout the day, you can identify trends that might otherwise go unnoticed.

For instance, if you document that high-sugar foods often lead to feelings of fatigue or a spike in blood sugar levels, you gain insights into how certain foods affect you. Similarly, tracking exercise routines alongside your energy levels can reveal which activities contribute most positively to your mood and health. This practice encourages mindful eating and exercising, fostering healthier habits over time.

Guideline: Start slow. Initially, record just one meal or activity per day, gradually building up to a comprehensive log. Reflect on this information weekly to identify patterns and make informed adjustments.

Mood Tracking: Emotional Awareness

Including mood tracking in your journal is another critical aspect of comprehensive diabetes management. Moods and emotions significantly influence daily decisions, including food choices and physical activity levels. Recognizing these emotional factors is vital in understanding their impact on your diabetes management.

By documenting how you feel at different times of the day, especially before and after meals or exercises, you can see how your emotions correlate with your behavior and health outcomes. For example, noticing a pattern of overeating when feeling stressed or anxious allows you to address these triggers proactively.

Guideline: Use a simple rating system or emojis to track moods. For instance, smiley faces for good moods, neutral faces for average feelings, and sad faces for negative emotions. This visual aid makes it easier to spot emotional patterns related to your habits.

Goal Setting and Reflection: Intentional Progress

Journals serve as a personal space to articulate goals and reflect on achievements, making the diabetes management process more intentional. Establishing clear, achievable goals helps maintain focus and motivation. Whether it's aiming for a specific blood sugar level, exercising a certain number of times per week, or reducing cravings for unhealthy food, setting these targets gives direction to your efforts.

Reflecting on your progress towards these goals is equally important. Regularly reviewing your journal entries can provide a sense of accomplishment and highlight areas needing improvement. Celebrating small victories motivates continued effort and reinforces the positive changes you've made.

Guideline: Write down both short-term and long-term goals in your journal. Reflect weekly or monthly on your achievements and challenges, adjusting your strategies as needed to stay on track.

Tracking Challenges: Documenting Setbacks and Solutions

Lastly, journaling about setbacks and finding solutions is essential for fostering resilience in diabetes management. No journey is without obstacles, and recognizing these hurdles early on allows for proactive problem-solving.

Documenting any difficulties you encounter, such as high blood sugar readings, skipped exercise sessions, or emotional eating episodes, helps identify recurring issues. Writing about these experiences not only provides an outlet for frustration but also initiates the search for practical solutions.

When tracking setbacks, consider what factors contributed to the problem. Was it a particularly stressful day? Did a change in routine throw off your usual schedule? Understanding the root causes enables you to strategize more effectively, whether by planning stress-relief activities, adjusting your diet, or modifying your exercise regimen.

Guideline: Keep a dedicated section in your journal for setbacks. Describe the issue, analyze potential triggers, and brainstorm possible solutions. Revisit this section periodically to track improvements and refine your strategies.

Practical Tips for Effective Journaling

1. **Consistency is Key:** Make journaling a daily habit, even if the entries are brief. Consistency ensures that you capture accurate and comprehensive data over time.
2. **Be Honest:** Record your true feelings and behaviors without judgment. Honesty in your entries will yield the most beneficial insights.
3. **Stay Organized:** Use sections or different notebooks for various aspects of your journaling, such as food intake, exercise, mood, goals, and setbacks. This organization makes it easier to review and analyze your records.
4. **Involve Your Care Team:** Share your journal with healthcare providers such as dietitians, therapists, or doctors. Their professional insights can help tailor your management plan to better fit your needs.

Guideline: Find a journaling method that works best for you. Whether it's a traditional notebook, a digital app, or even voice recordings, choose a medium that feels comfortable and is easy to maintain.

Conclusion

Effective journaling is a multifaceted approach that can significantly enhance diabetes management. By logging daily behaviors, tracking mood, articulating goals, and documenting setbacks, individuals with diabetes can gain insightful perspectives into their habits and health. This process not only aids in better managing diabetes but also promotes a more intentional and resilient approach to overall well-being.

Technology Aids Like Apps and Devices

Advancements in technology have revolutionized the way seniors can manage their health, particularly for those managing diabetes. With an array of tools and resources available, seniors can effectively track essential health parameters and monitor the formation of healthy habits. By utilizing accessible apps, wearable devices, online support communities, and educational resources, they can take greater control over their well-being.

Firstly, health-monitoring apps have emerged as user-friendly solutions that allow seniors to track various aspects of their health. These apps often include features such as tracking nutrition, exercise, and blood sugar levels. For instance, apps like MyFitnessPal or Carb Manager enable users to log their daily food intake, which is crucial for managing diabetes. By monitoring what they eat, seniors can understand the impact of different foods on their blood sugar levels and receive personalized dietary recommendations (*Health-Monitoring Devices and Apps for Seniors*, 2024).

Exercise tracking is another significant feature found in many health-monitoring apps. Applications like Fitbit or Apple Health provide seniors with the ability to record their physical activities, such as steps taken, distance covered, and calories burned. This information can help them stay motivated and maintain a consistent exercise regimen, which is vital for managing diabetes. Additionally, apps dedicated to tracking blood sugar levels, such as Glucose Buddy, allow seniors to log their readings and track trends over time, providing valuable insights into their condition.

Transitioning to wearable technology, fitness trackers and continuous glucose monitors (CGMs) serve as powerful tools for seniors. Fitness trackers like Fitbit or Garmin are worn on the wrist, offering real-time data on physical activity. These devices can track steps, heart rate, sleep patterns, and even remind users to move if they've been sedentary for too long. Such information encourages seniors to stay active and helps in maintaining an overall healthy lifestyle.

Continuous glucose monitors, on the other hand, provide real-time blood sugar measurements through a sensor placed under the skin. Devices like the FreeStyle Libre or Dexcom CGM continuously monitor glucose levels, sending alerts to the user's smartphone if their levels go too high or too low (The Best Wearable Technology for Seniors with Diabetes, 2024). This not only aids in better blood glucose management but also reduces the need for finger-prick tests, making it easier for seniors with limited manual dexterity to manage their diabetes.

In addition to individual tracking, online platforms and communities play a crucial role in enhancing motivation and accountability. Websites and forums such as Diabetic Connect or TuDiabetes allow seniors to share their experiences, ask questions, and seek advice from others facing similar challenges. Engaging with these communities fosters a sense of belonging and support, encouraging seniors to stick to their health goals.

Moreover, many health-monitoring apps and platforms offer incentive programs where users can earn rewards or badges for reaching specific milestones. This gamification of health tracking can be particularly motivating, as it adds an element of fun and competition. Caregivers and family members can also participate by creating shared goals and celebrating achievements together, further reinforcing positive behavior.

Another indispensable resource for seniors is the variety of educational tools available online. Websites such as the American Diabetes Association and the National Institute on Aging provide a wealth of information on managing diabetes, including articles, videos, and webinars. These resources cover topics such as understanding blood sugar levels, meal planning, and the importance of regular exercise.

Additionally, some platforms offer interactive elements, like virtual workshops or live Q&A sessions with healthcare professionals. These opportunities enable seniors to deepen their knowledge and stay informed about the latest advancements in diabetes management. For instance, online courses or webinars on topics like "Improving Your Diet" or "Staying Active with Diabetes" can provide practical tips and strategies that seniors can implement in their daily lives.

For those who prefer a more structured approach, specialized programs like Diabetes Self-Management Education and Support (DSMES) offer comprehensive guidance. These programs typically run in-person or online and cover various aspects of diabetes care, including medication management, coping strategies, and preventive measures. Participating in such programs can be highly beneficial, as they offer personalized feedback and support from certified educators.

Furthermore, many seniors benefit from using combination approaches that integrate multiple technologies. For example, a senior might use a fitness tracker to monitor their physical activity, a CGM to keep track of their blood sugar levels, and a health-monitoring app to log their meals and medications. By consolidating data from different sources, they can get a holistic view of their health, making it easier to identify patterns and make informed decisions.

When adopting these technologies, it's important to consider ease of use and accessibility. User-friendly designs with large, clear displays and intuitive navigation are essential for seniors who may not be tech-savvy. Customizable settings that allow adjustments to font size, color schemes, and notification preferences can also enhance usability (*Health-Monitoring Devices and Apps for Seniors*, 2024). Ensuring privacy and security features are in place is equally important, especially when dealing with sensitive health information.

Celebrating Milestones and Progress

Recognizing and Celebrating Achievements

When managing diabetes, recognizing and celebrating achievements in habit tracking is crucial for keeping motivation high and sustaining commitment over the long term. Celebrations can range from small acknowledgments of daily successes to larger rewards for significant milestones. The act of recognition itself keeps individuals engaged and excited about their progress, a key factor often overlooked in habit formation.

Setting and Acknowledging Personal Milestones

Personal milestones are essential markers that indicate progress in diabetes management. These milestones could be as simple as maintaining a steady blood sugar level for a week or as significant as achieving a target weight. To set these milestones effectively, it's important to make them specific and realistic. For instance, instead of setting a vague goal like "improve diet," aim for something more concrete such as "include at least one serving of vegetables in each meal."

Once milestones are defined, acknowledging them becomes the next critical step. This can be accomplished through various means—writing down the achievements in a journal, sharing them with a close friend, or even marking them on a calendar. Acknowledgment serves as a constant reminder of the journey embarked upon and the progress made, reinforcing positive behavior and commitment. Recognizing effort fuels the desire to continue, creating a cycle of ongoing improvement.

Creating Reward Systems

A well-structured reward system can provide additional motivation to pursue and achieve set milestones. Rewards don't have to be extravagant; they just need to be meaningful to the individual. Practical rewards might include a favorite activity, a small gift, or a special outing. For seniors, a reward could be something relaxing and enjoyable, like a visit to a favorite park or a day spent with grandchildren.

To set up a practical reward system, start by identifying what types of rewards would be most motivating. Incorporate a mix of short-term and long-term rewards. Short-term rewards could be something immediate, like enjoying a favorite hobby after a successful week of tracking habits. Long-term rewards might be a planned vacation or a new piece of fitness equipment after maintaining healthy habits for several months. This combination helps maintain interest and provides continuous motivation.

Encouraging Seniors to Share Successes

Sharing achievements with family members or support groups can significantly enhance a sense of community and belonging. It also provides an added layer of accountability. When others are aware of goals and progress, it creates an external motivation to stay on track. Health is often a family affair, and involving loved ones can make the journey easier and more enjoyable.

Encourage seniors to communicate their milestones and successes regularly. This can be done in person, over the phone, or through social media groups dedicated to health and wellness. Support groups, whether local or online, offer a platform to share stories, celebrate victories, and receive encouragement during challenging times. The act of sharing not only boosts the morale of the individual but can also inspire others within the community to strive towards their own health goals.

Strategies for Maintaining Motivation

Maintaining motivation after reaching a milestone can sometimes be challenging. However, there are several strategies to keep the momentum going. One effective approach is to continuously set new, achievable goals. As soon as one milestone is reached, identify another target to work towards. This ongoing goal-setting creates a sense of purpose and direction, preventing feelings of stagnation.

Another strategy is to reflect on the journey so far. Keeping a journal where thoughts, feelings, and experiences related to diabetes management are recorded can be incredibly therapeutic. Reflect on what has been accomplished, the challenges overcome, and the lessons learned along the way. This reflection fosters a deeper understanding of personal growth and the value of the hard work invested.

Visual representations of achievements can also play a significant role in maintaining motivation. Charts or graphs showing progress in blood sugar levels, weight loss, or physical activities serve as tangible evidence of improvements. Regularly updating and reviewing these visual tools can reinforce the sense that efforts are yielding results.

Flexibility and adjustments are equally important. Be prepared to modify goals and reward systems as needed. If a particular milestone seems consistently out of reach, reassess its feasibility and make necessary adjustments. Conversely, if goals are too easily achieved, consider setting slightly more challenging targets to ensure continued progress and engagement.

Finally, celebrate non-scale victories. While numerical metrics like weight and blood sugar levels are important, other forms of progress should also be acknowledged. Improved energy levels, better sleep quality, enhanced mood, and increased stamina are all significant achievements worth celebrating. These non-scale victories contribute to overall well-being and provide additional reassurance that positive changes are happening.

Conclusion

Final Thoughts

Regularly tracking habits and health improvements plays a vital role in managing diabetes, particularly for seniors. This chapter has emphasized the importance of monitoring daily activities such as diet, exercise, and medication adherence. By doing so, seniors can gain valuable insights into how specific habits affect their blood sugar levels and overall health. Understanding these patterns empowers them to make informed decisions, leading to better glycemic control and increased motivation to maintain healthy behaviors. Furthermore, sharing this data with healthcare providers or caregivers adds an extra layer of accountability, ensuring that seniors remain committed to their health goals.

The benefits of habit tracking extend beyond just physical health; they also offer psychological advantages. Visible progress, illustrated through graphs and logs, provides tangible proof of efforts paying off, boosting confidence and maintaining long-term commitment. Technology, like Continuous Glucose Monitoring systems and health apps, has made tracking more accessible and effective by providing real-time feedback and personalized recommendations. These advancements simplify the management process, making it less overwhelming and more manageable for seniors. Overall, consistent tracking and the use of supportive tools create a proactive approach to diabetes management, fostering a healthier and more engaged lifestyle.

9

Staying Motivated: Overcoming Challenges

Staying motivated is key to managing diabetes effectively. It's natural to face challenges and setbacks along this journey, but they don't define your ability to succeed. Rather than viewing obstacles as insurmountable, embracing them as part of the process can lead to personal growth and improved health outcomes.

This chapter delves into practical strategies for maintaining motivation and overcoming common hurdles in habit formation. You'll explore techniques like setting realistic goals, practicing self-compassion, and reflecting on past experiences to extract valuable lessons. By understanding that setbacks are a normal part of the journey, you can develop a resilient mindset and stay focused on your long-term health objectives. Through real-life examples and actionable advice, this chapter aims to equip you with the tools needed to navigate the ups and downs of diabetes management with confidence and determination.

Dealing with Setbacks

Navigating setbacks is an inevitable part of life, especially when managing diabetes. Understanding that these obstacles are normal and learning practical strategies to effectively handle them can make the journey less daunting. Here, we delve into the importance of recognizing setbacks, practicing self-compassion, outlining actionable steps, and extracting valuable lessons from these experiences.

Firstly, it's crucial to recognize that setbacks happen to everyone. Whether you're newly diagnosed or have been managing diabetes for years, experiencing setbacks is a common occurrence. It's easy to feel isolated or discouraged when facing challenges, but understanding that others share similar struggles can provide comfort and alleviate some of the stress. Acknowledging that setbacks are part of the process helps normalize the experience and reduces feelings of isolation. When you see your journey as part of a collective human experience, it's easier to remain resilient and focused on your goals.

Self-compassion plays a vital role during these challenging times. Instead of viewing setbacks as failures, consider them opportunities for growth. Practicing self-compassion involves treating yourself with kindness and understanding rather than harsh judgment. By doing so, you can build emotional resilience, which allows you to bounce back more quickly from difficulties. As noted by Andrea Zorbas in her exploration of self-compassion, this approach not only improves mental health by reducing anxiety and depression but also enhances relationships and personal growth (The, 2024). This shift in perspective enables you to maintain motivation and continue on your path despite temporary setbacks.

When setbacks occur, it's essential to take proactive steps to address them. Start by reassessing your goals. Were they too ambitious or not aligned with your current capabilities? Adjusting your goals to be more realistic can prevent future discouragement. Next, identify any triggers that may have contributed to the setback. For example, if you notice that stress leads to poor dietary choices, you can implement stress-management techniques such as meditation or gentle exercise. Creating a list of potential triggers and developing strategies to mitigate them can significantly improve your ability to stay on track.

Moreover, reflecting on each setback offers valuable insights into your personal habits and triggers. Take some time to think about what went wrong and why. What external factors influenced your behavior? How did your internal mindset affect your choices? By analyzing these elements, you can learn more about yourself and develop better coping mechanisms for the future. This reflection process turns setbacks into powerful learning experiences rather than mere obstacles.

For instance, let's consider the story of Margaret, a senior living with diabetes. She found that her blood sugar levels would spike whenever she attended family gatherings, where temptation to indulge in sweets was high. Initially, she felt frustrated and blamed herself for lack of discipline. Over time, however, she adopted a compassionate approach. Margaret started bringing healthy snacks to gatherings and practiced mindful eating. She also communicated her needs with family members, who supported her efforts by offering healthier options. Through reassessment and the application of self-compassion, she turned her setback into a stepping stone for better management of her diabetes.

Additionally, it's important to integrate mindfulness into your approach to setbacks. Mindfulness involves being present and fully aware of your thoughts and emotions without over-identifying with them. This practice can help you observe negative patterns and respond to them more thoughtfully. For example, if a setback makes you feel overwhelmed, mindfulness can help you recognize this feeling without letting it dominate your actions. Instead of reacting impulsively, you can choose more constructive responses that align with your long-term goals.

Another strategy to navigate setbacks is to foster a strong support network. Surround yourself with people who understand your journey and can offer encouragement. This could include family members, friends, caregivers, or support groups. Sharing your experiences and hearing others' stories can provide new perspectives and reinforce the notion that you are not alone in your struggles. Furthermore, health professionals can offer tailored advice and resources to help you overcome specific challenges related to diabetes management.

Consider the case of John, a patient who struggled to maintain physical activity due to joint pain. His initial attempts to exercise resulted in increased discomfort, leading him to abandon his regimen altogether. Feeling defeated, he spoke to his healthcare provider, who suggested low-impact activities like swimming or yoga. With the support and guidance of his healthcare team, John gradually incorporated these exercises into his routine and experienced significant improvements in his overall health. His story highlights the importance of seeking professional advice and adapting strategies to fit individual needs.

Strategies to Stay Motivated

Maintaining motivation in the face of challenges is crucial for effective diabetes management and overall well-being. This section aims to equip readers with actionable strategies that can help sustain their motivation, even when obstacles arise.

Setting SMART (Specific, Measurable, Achievable, Relevant, Time-bound) goals is a critical first step. SMART goals offer a structured approach to setting objectives, making them easier to achieve. For instance, instead of setting a vague goal like "improving diet," aim for more specific targets such as "eating five servings of vegetables each day." Measuring progress becomes simpler, allowing individuals to track their success. Measurable goals also provide a sense of accomplishment, reinforcing motivation. It's important that these goals are achievable and suited to individual lifestyles. For seniors managing diabetes, an example might be scheduling 30 minutes of light exercise, such as walking or stretching, three times a week. Ensuring goals are relevant helps maintain focus, and having time-bound deadlines prevents procrastination, adding a sense of urgency and purpose.

Connecting habits to personal values or life goals can significantly boost intrinsic motivation. When habits resonate with deeper values, they feel more meaningful and less like chores. For example, if family is a core value, think about how managing diabetes effectively allows for more quality time with loved ones. Visualizing long-term benefits, like staying healthy to attend a grandchild's graduation, can drive daily actions. Engaging in activities that align with core values makes it easier to adhere to new habits, reducing resistance and increasing commitment.

Utilizing visual reminders, such as vision boards or planning apps, can keep motivation levels high. Vision boards can be a collection of images and quotes that represent personal goals and aspirations. Creating one can be a fun and engaging activity that provides a daily visual cue to stay on track. Planning apps, on the other hand, offer practical functionality by helping to schedule tasks and set reminders. For tech-savvy seniors, using a smartphone app to track blood sugar levels or log meals can be tremendously helpful. Regular notifications serve as prompts, keeping health management at the forefront of daily routines.

Cultivating positive self-talk through affirmations and surrounding oneself with positive influences is another essential strategy. Positive self-talk involves countering negative thoughts with encouraging and affirming language. Simple phrases like "I am capable of managing my health" or "Every small step counts" can foster a constructive mindset. This practice can be further reinforced by reading inspirational stories or quotes regularly. Surrounding oneself with a supportive network also plays a vital role in maintaining motivation. Family members, friends, and community groups can offer encouragement and share successes, making the journey less lonely. Being part of a support group where individuals have similar health goals can provide emotional sustenance and practical advice.

While pursuing these strategies, it's crucial to remember the importance of adaptability and flexibility. Life is unpredictable, and setbacks are inevitable. Maintaining motivation requires an ability to reassess and adjust goals as needed. For instance, if a planned exercise routine becomes too strenuous, it's okay to switch to a gentler activity. Flexibility not only prevents burnout but also keeps the journey enjoyable and sustainable in the long term.

In addition, it's beneficial to break down larger goals into smaller, manageable tasks. Tackling large objectives can be overwhelming, leading to discouragement. Micro-actions make big ambitions more approachable. If the aim is to incorporate more physical activity, start with short ten-minute walks and build up gradually. Each small win builds momentum, contributing to the ultimate goal without feeling daunting. This methodical approach ensures steady progress, keeping motivation alive.

Furthermore, keeping a wellness journal can be an excellent way to document progress and stay motivated. Writing down daily achievements, no matter how small, provides a visual representation of progress and serves as a reminder of one's capabilities. Reflecting on these entries can reignite motivation during challenging times. Noting patterns and triggers in the journal can also provide insights, enabling better management of routines and habits.

Lastly, seek professional guidance when necessary. Healthcare professionals, wellness coaches, or therapists can offer tailored advice, addressing specific challenges and providing personalized strategies. They can ensure that habits and goals are medically sound and aligned with individual health needs. Professional input can add an extra layer of support, offering both accountability and expertise.

In summary, maintaining motivation amidst challenges involves a multifaceted approach: setting SMART goals, connecting habits to personal values, utilizing visual reminders, fostering positive self-talk, embracing flexibility, breaking down ambitions into micro-actions, documenting progress, and seeking professional guidance. Each strategy contributes to sustaining motivation, making the path to effective diabetes management and overall well-being more achievable and less daunting.

Real-life Success Stories

Inspiring readers through relatable stories of individuals who have successfully navigated their diabetes journey can provide a powerful source of motivation and hope. Sharing diverse success stories that highlight unique approaches to managing diabetes enables readers to see possibilities tailored to their individual circumstances.

Consider Maggie, a 65-year-old grandmother who discovered she had type 2 diabetes five years ago. Initially overwhelmed by the diagnosis, Maggie found solace and guidance in joining a local diabetes support group. Through the group's collective wisdom, she learned how to integrate diabetes management into her daily routine seamlessly. Maggie's approach involved pairing blood glucose monitoring with her morning and evening tooth brushing, a strategy recommended by health professionals (Hood et al., 2019). This small habit became a cornerstone of her daily routine and helped maintain consistent monitoring without feeling burdensome.

Similarly, John, a retired teacher, approached his diabetes management uniquely. John's passion for gardening served as a therapeutic outlet and doubled as a form of physical activity. By dedicating an hour each day to tending his garden, John not only enjoyed a sense of peace but also maintained regular exercise. This small but consistent habit translated into significant life changes, illustrating how persistent actions create major impacts over time.

Another compelling story is that of Ella, a 70-year-old retiree who took a scientific route to understanding her condition. Ella embraced continuous glucose monitoring (CGM) technology, which provided real-time information on her blood glucose levels. By using CGM, Ella could make timely adjustments to her insulin dosages, optimizing her glycemic control (Sugandh et al., 2023). This data-driven method allowed her greater autonomy and precision in managing her diabetes, showcasing how modern technology can empower individuals in their health journeys.

Lessons learned from these journeys underline the importance of persistence, curiosity, and experimentation. Maggie's story emphasizes persistence. Despite initial setbacks, she remained committed to finding a manageable routine, demonstrating that long-term success often hinges on staying dedicated even when progress seems slow. John's tale highlights curiosity—his willingness to explore how his love for gardening could benefit his health opened new avenues for integrating physical activity into his life. Ella's experience underscores the value of experimentation. By trying out different technologies and methods, she found a system that worked best for her, proving that personalized approaches can yield better outcomes.

Social support and community play crucial roles in achieving health goals, as illustrated in these narratives. Maggie's participation in a support group provided emotional reinforcement and practical advice, fostering a sense of belonging and accountability. For John, the encouragement from fellow gardeners in his community motivated him to stay active and engaged. Similarly, Ella's involvement in online forums where users discussed CGM technologies offered her a platform to share challenges and successes, reinforcing her commitment to effective diabetes management.

These stories collectively stress the importance of having a support system for accountability and encouragement. Developing a personal plan to reassess goals and identify triggers is vital in navigating diabetes management. Routine check-ins, either with healthcare providers or within support groups, can help evaluate feelings and adjust strategies as necessary.

The benefits of social support are evident in the positive outcomes experienced by these individuals. Establishing a network of family, friends, and healthcare professionals who provide regular reinforcement when diabetes management behaviors are completed can significantly enhance adherence to treatment plans (Hood et al., 2019).

Furthermore, these narratives impart valuable lessons for caregivers and health professionals working with seniors. Understanding the diversity of approaches that can lead to successful diabetes management allows them to offer more personalized and relatable advice. Encouraging patients to find small habits that fit into their daily routines, such as Maggie's integration of glucose monitoring with tooth brushing, can make management feel less intrusive and more sustainable.

Caregivers can play a supportive role by helping their loved ones craft and maintain these small yet impactful habits. For instance, they can assist in setting up reminders or helping organize a comfortable space for activities like gardening, akin to John's routine. Providing moral support and acknowledging the efforts put into maintaining these habits can boost motivation and reinforce the individual's commitment to their health goals.

Health professionals, on the other hand, should promote the usage of tools like CGM for those inclined towards technological solutions. Educating patients about the availability and benefits of such advancements can equip them with better tools for self-management. Additionally, promoting the formation of or participation in support groups can be incredibly beneficial, as seen with Maggie's success.

Turning Obstacles into Opportunities

Challenges and obstacles are inevitable in the journey towards effective diabetes management, especially for seniors trying to form new habits. However, it is crucial to understand that these challenges are not insurmountable barriers but opportunities for growth. Shifting our perspective can empower us to overcome difficulties with resilience and determination.

One fundamental approach to viewing challenges positively is by adopting a growth mindset. The concept of a growth mindset, pioneered by psychologist Carol Dweck, revolves around the belief that intelligence and abilities can be developed through dedication and hard work rather than being fixed traits. This mindset encourages individuals to see setbacks not as failures but as valuable learning experiences. For seniors managing diabetes, this means understanding that every obstacle encountered offers a chance to improve and refine their approach to a healthier lifestyle (Jagtiani, 2024).

Embracing a growth mindset involves seeing each challenge as an opportunity to develop new skills or strengthen existing ones. For example, if a senior struggles to maintain a balanced diet due to a lack of knowledge about healthy foods, this challenge presents an opportunity to learn more about nutrition. Attending workshops, consulting with a dietitian, or even exploring reliable online resources can provide the necessary information and turn a perceived barrier into a stepping stone towards better health.

A proactive approach to problem-solving is essential when facing challenges. This involves re-evaluating the obstacles and identifying potential areas for growth. For instance, if managing blood sugar levels becomes difficult due to irregular meal timings, one could re-assess their daily schedule and find ways to prioritize consistent eating habits. Perhaps setting reminders or planning meals in advance can help streamline this process. By addressing the root causes of the challenges, it becomes easier to develop practical solutions that contribute to long-term improvement.

Flexibility is another key factor in overcoming obstacles. Adopting flexible strategies allows individuals to adapt their methods based on what works best for them personally. Suppose a particular exercise routine proves too strenuous or unenjoyable; instead of giving up, one could explore alternative forms of physical activity such as walking, swimming, or yoga. The willingness to adjust and experiment with different approaches ensures that setbacks do not derail progress but rather lead to discovering methods that are both effective and enjoyable.

Persistence plays a critical role in surmounting challenges. It's important to recognize that persistence does not mean relentlessly pushing forward without reflection. Instead, it involves a continuous cycle of trying, evaluating, learning, and adapting. Seniors managing diabetes can benefit from documenting their personal victories, no matter how small. Keeping a journal to track daily achievements, like maintaining consistent blood sugar levels or successfully resisting unhealthy food cravings, can provide both motivation and a tangible record of progress. Celebrating these successes reinforces a positive outlook and fosters a sense of accomplishment.

To further illustrate the power of persistence, consider a scenario where a senior faces difficulty adhering to a prescribed medication regimen. They might struggle with remembering to take their medications or feel overwhelmed by the number of pills. By acknowledging the challenge and seeking solutions, such as using a pill organizer or setting alarms, they can gradually develop a routine that fits seamlessly into their daily life. Persistently working towards integrating this routine can lead to significant improvements in their overall health management.

Encouraging seniors to write down what each setback teaches them about their personal habits or triggers is a valuable practice. For instance, if a senior notices that stress leads to poor dietary choices, they can identify stress management techniques to mitigate this trigger. Documenting these insights helps build self-awareness and informs future decisions, ultimately contributing to better habit formation and diabetes management.

Final Insights

Managing diabetes is a journey that inevitably includes challenges. This chapter has emphasized the importance of recognizing setbacks as a natural part of this process and learning to approach them with self-compassion and practical strategies. By understanding that obstacles are common, practicing kindness towards yourself, and reassessing goals when needed, you can maintain motivation and continue progressing. Embracing mindfulness, building a support network, and reflecting on experiences turn setbacks into valuable learning opportunities, helping you adapt and grow stronger in your diabetes management.

The stories and examples provided highlight that perseverance, flexibility, and support are key factors in overcoming hurdles. Whether it's through personal reflection, adjusting daily routines, or seeking help from professionals and loved ones, each step taken strengthens your ability to manage diabetes effectively. Remember that every challenge faced is an opportunity for growth. By staying committed and compassionate towards yourself, you can transform obstacles into stepping stones, making your journey toward health and well-being more achievable and rewarding.

10

Sustaining Healthy Habits: Long-Term Success

Sustaining healthy habits is a matter of integrating them into your daily life in ways that feel natural and manageable. For many, the key to lasting change lies in embedding these habits smoothly into existing routines, making it less likely that they'll be forgotten or abandoned over time. This chapter will guide you through practical methods designed to make new behaviors a regular part of your day-to-day activities, providing strategies tailored specifically for seniors, caregivers, and health professionals.

Throughout this chapter, you'll explore various approaches to ensuring these healthy habits stick. You'll learn about "habit stacking," a technique that involves pairing new habits with established ones to create seamless transitions. We will also delve into the power of environmental cues and how small adjustments in your surroundings can lead to significant improvements in behavior. Additionally, the importance of routine check-ins and self-reflection will be highlighted as essential tools for tracking progress and maintaining motivation. Finally, we'll discuss the significance of flexibility within routines, allowing you to adapt to life's inevitable changes while staying committed to your goals. By following these steps, you can create a sustainable path toward long-term health and well-being.

Embedding habits into daily routines

Integrating new habits into existing routines is a powerful strategy for ensuring long-term success in sustaining healthy behaviors. This approach not only reinforces consistency but also makes it easier to adopt and maintain new habits over time.

Habit Stacking

Habit stacking is an effective method that simplifies daily life by incorporating new habits into already established routines. Imagine you want to start taking vitamins every morning but keep forgetting. One way to solve this is by placing your vitamins next to the coffee machine if having coffee is part of your daily routine. By doing this, you create a natural trigger — as soon as you make your coffee, you'll be reminded to take your vitamins. This method allows new habits to become a seamless part of your day.

For instance, consider someone who exercises regularly but often skips stretching afterward. They could stack the habit of stretching immediately after their workout session since they are already in the mindset of physical activity. This sequence makes it less likely to forget the new habit because it rides on the coattails of an existing one. Essentially, the established habit acts as a cue for initiating the new behavior, making the integration process more intuitive and less obtrusive to your daily schedule.

Environmental Cues

Another critical aspect of embedding new habits into your life involves modifying your environment. Strategic placement of reminders can significantly influence the likelihood of engaging in positive behaviors without requiring conscious effort. For example, individuals aiming to stay hydrated might place water bottles in various frequently visited spots around their home. Seeing these water bottles throughout the day serves as a constant visual reminder to drink more water.

Similarly, those wanting to eat healthier snacks can keep fruits or nuts in easily accessible places while storing less healthy options out of sight. This small environmental change can make a significant impact on one's choices. Adjusting your physical environment can subtly guide your actions, making the adoption of new habits more natural and automatic.

Routine Check-Ins and Self-Reflection

Integrating new habits isn't merely about environmental tweaks or stacking habits; it also requires regular self-reflection and check-ins to evaluate progress and maintain motivation. Routine check-ins offer a structured way to assess whether the new habits are effectively merging with your lifestyle or if adjustments are needed. For instance, setting aside time each week to reflect on your progress can help identify what's working and what might need modification.

These sessions of self-reflection should focus on both successes and obstacles. Celebrate small victories to reinforce positive behavior and analyze any difficulties to develop strategies for overcoming them. This reflective practice ensures that you remain conscious of your goals and committed to achieving them, making it easier to stay on track over the long term.

Flexibility in Routines

Finally, flexibility within routines is crucial for long-term success in maintaining new habits. Life is full of unexpected changes, and rigid routines can quickly become unmanageable when circumstances shift. Therefore, it's essential to build flexibility into your routines, allowing you to adjust habits based on changing circumstances without feeling discouraged.

For instance, you might have a habit of walking in the park every morning. However, on days when the weather is bad, you could switch to an indoor exercise like yoga instead. This flexibility ensures that you continue engaging in beneficial activities even when your original plan isn't feasible. It prevents disruptions from derailing your efforts and helps you adapt to new situations while sticking to your overall objective of leading a healthier life.

By recognizing the importance of adaptability, you empower yourself to sustain new habits through various stages and changes in life. Flexibility doesn't mean being inconsistent; rather, it means being resilient and resourceful in how you achieve your goals.

Reflecting on benefits and progress

Recognizing and appreciating the positive changes engendered by new habits is integral to sustaining those habits over time. This subpoint will detail practical strategies to foster gratitude, visualize progress, celebrate milestones, and engage in mindful reflection sessions. These approaches not only reinforce positive behaviors but also provide a continuous source of motivation for maintaining healthy habits.

Introducing gratitude practices can play a pivotal role in enhancing motivation. One effective method is journaling about the benefits experienced from newly adopted habits. Writing down daily or weekly reflections on how these changes are making a difference can serve as a powerful reminder of why you started. For instance, if regular exercise has led to improved blood sugar levels and increased energy, noting these improvements helps reinforce the commitment to staying active. This practice aligns with the findings that expressing gratitude can significantly boost overall happiness and well-being (Chapter 28. Spirituality and Community Building | Section 9. Gratitude and Appreciation | Main Section | Community Tool Box, n.d.).

Creating visual representations of progress, such as charts and graphs, can make accomplishments tangible and exciting. By tracking your progress in a visible format, you create a constant reminder of how far you've come. For seniors managing diabetes, this could mean plotting blood glucose levels on a graph or marking off days on a calendar where they adhered to their dietary plans. Visual aids serve as a motivational tool, making it easier to see patterns of improvement and providing a sense of achievement. Engaging family members in creating these visuals can also turn it into a collaborative effort, strengthening support systems and making health management a shared activity.

Celebrating milestones is crucial for reinforcing positive behavior. Setting specific goals and acknowledging when they are achieved can foster a sense of accomplishment. These milestones don't have to be monumental; even small victories like consistently taking medication on time or integrating a new type of vegetable into your diet are worth celebrating. Personal recognition might involve treating yourself to a favorite activity or indulgence, while group recognition can include sharing successes in support groups or family gatherings. This collective celebration further solidifies the habit, as the positive reinforcement from peers and loved ones can be highly motivating.

Encouraging mindful reflection sessions allows for periodic evaluation of what's working and what's not, fostering ongoing motivation. Taking time to sit quietly and reflect on recent experiences can help identify areas of improvement and acknowledge progress. This mindful approach not only facilitates self-awareness but also provides opportunities to adjust strategies as needed. For example, if a particular exercise routine isn't producing desired results, reflecting on this can prompt a change to something more effective and enjoyable. Mindful reflection ensures that the journey towards healthier habits remains flexible and tailored to individual needs, promoting sustained engagement.

Future planning for sustained health

Planning for continued health management in the years to come is crucial, particularly for seniors managing diabetes. By establishing specific, measurable, and personalized long-term health goals, seniors can ensure a higher quality of life and sustained health. One effective guideline for setting these goals involves using the SMART criteria: goals should be Specific, Measurable, Achievable, Relevant, and Time-bound.

For example, instead of a general goal like "I want to feel healthier," a more effective goal would be "I will walk for 30 minutes every day for the next month." This goal is specific (walking), measurable (30 minutes daily), achievable (adaptable based on current fitness level), relevant (improves cardiovascular health), and time-bound (one month). Seniors may benefit from using planning tools such as daily journals or health apps that are specifically adapted for their needs, allowing them to track progress and make adjustments as needed.

Integrating regular medical assessments into daily habits is another critical strategy. Regular check-ups can help manage and monitor diabetes effectively. Routine examinations should include blood pressure checks, cholesterol assessments, and eye exams to catch potential complications early. For instance, having systematic yearly kidney function tests can prevent severe consequences related to diabetes. Developing a habit of scheduling and attending these appointments ensures continuous monitoring and timely intervention.

Seniors should also make use of technology by setting reminders on their phones or using paper calendars prominently displayed at home. This approach helps create a routine around medical assessments, turning them into an integral part of their lifestyle rather than a disruptive chore.

Continuous education on diabetes management plays a pivotal role in maintaining health. Staying informed about the latest treatments, dietary guidelines, and self-care practices can empower seniors to take control of their condition. For instance, subscribing to reputable newsletters or joining online communities devoted to diabetes management provides ongoing information and peer support. Continuous education enables seniors to adapt to new findings and incorporate them into their health management plans, ensuring they remain proactive rather than reactive regarding their health.

Ongoing education can take many forms, including attending seminars hosted by healthcare providers, subscribing to informational publications, or participating in workshops. These resources provide updates on advancements in diabetes care and management, new medications, and lifestyle modifications.

Building a sustainable support system is equally vital. Joining support groups allows seniors to share experiences and coping strategies with others who understand their challenges. This sense of community can reduce feelings of isolation and provide emotional support. Identifying supportive friends and family members who can offer encouragement and practical help is essential. These individuals can accompany seniors to medical appointments, assist with meal planning, or simply provide companionship during exercise routines.

A practical guideline for establishing a support network includes reaching out to local senior centers or healthcare providers for recommendations on support groups. Additionally, many communities offer programs specifically designed for seniors with diabetes, providing tailored resources and a welcoming environment.

Support systems can extend beyond personal relationships to include professional assistance. Dietitians, diabetes educators, and mental health professionals can offer invaluable guidance and support, addressing specific needs related to diet, stress management, and overall well-being. Utilizing these resources ensures a comprehensive approach to diabetes management that addresses both physical and emotional health.

Managing diabetes successfully requires a multi-faceted approach that includes setting realistic long-term goals, integrating regular medical assessments, staying informed through continuous education, and building robust support networks. By following these strategies, seniors can manage their diabetes more effectively and enjoy a healthier, more fulfilling life.

As part of the process, it's essential to outline specific, measurable steps. For example, setting milestones such as scheduling quarterly doctors' visits, attending monthly support group meetings, and participating in weekly educational webinars on diabetes management. These actionable steps provide a clear roadmap and help maintain focus on long-term health objectives.

Moreover, integrating healthy habits into daily routines can bolster overall health. Small changes, like incorporating more vegetables into meals or choosing whole grains over processed foods, can have significant cumulative effects. Exercise, such as incorporating strength training or yoga sessions, not only aids in blood sugar control but also enhances mobility and mental clarity.

In addition, seniors should prioritize mental well-being alongside physical health. Engaging in hobbies, spending time with loved ones, and practicing mindfulness or meditation can significantly reduce stress and promote a positive outlook. Managing stress is particularly important for those with diabetes, as high-stress levels can adversely affect blood sugar levels.

Lastly, it is crucial to maintain open communication with healthcare providers. Seniors should feel empowered to discuss any concerns or difficulties in managing their diabetes, whether related to medication side effects, financial constraints, or lifestyle adjustments. Open dialogue allows for personalized care plans that cater to individual needs and circumstances.

Leaving a legacy of wellness

As we embark on the journey of sustaining healthy habits, it is crucial to not only focus on personal well-being but also consider the impact these habits can have on future generations. By embracing and sharing healthy living practices, seniors can create a legacy of wellness that positively affects their families and communities. Here are some practical ways to make this vision a reality.

Engaging in knowledge-sharing with family and friends is a powerful way to act as mentors in healthy living. This can be done through regular conversations about health topics, sharing tips on diet, exercise, and stress management, and even demonstrating healthy habits during family gatherings. When seniors take the lead in adopting and promoting healthy behaviors, they inspire younger generations to follow suit. Sharing stories of personal health improvements, challenges faced, and the strategies used to overcome them can provide invaluable guidance and motivation for others. By becoming active communicators of health knowledge, seniors can lay the foundation for a healthier family culture that transcends generations.

Involving family in healthy habits through joint activities is another effective approach. For instance, exercising together as a family not only promotes physical fitness but also strengthens familial bonds. Activities like walking, cycling, or participating in group sports can be enjoyable for all ages and create lasting memories. Cooking healthy meals together is another wonderful opportunity to teach and learn. Seniors can share their culinary skills and knowledge about nutritious food choices, while younger family members may introduce new recipes or cooking techniques. This shared experience fosters not only a love for healthy eating but also a deeper appreciation for spending time together.

Mindful meditations are yet another activity that can be practiced collectively. Regular meditation sessions can help reduce stress, improve mental clarity, and enhance emotional well-being. Seniors can guide their families through simple meditation exercises, creating a calm and supportive environment where everyone feels connected and at peace. These practices model positive coping mechanisms and self-care routines, which are essential for long-term health.

Documenting healthy choices through a journal or blog serves multiple purposes. Firstly, it provides a personal record of one's health journey, including successes, setbacks, and learning experiences. This documentation can offer valuable insights and reflections that help maintain motivation and track progress. Secondly, it becomes a resource for others. Family members, friends, or even a broader audience if shared online, can benefit from this repository of knowledge and experience. It ensures that lessons learned are not lost but rather preserved and accessible to those who seek guidance on their own paths to wellness.

Journaling can include various elements such as meal plans, exercise routines, meditation practices, and personal reflections. Over time, this compilation of information can become a comprehensive guide that others can refer to when looking for practical advice or inspiration. Additionally, maintaining a blog can facilitate interaction with a wider community of like-minded individuals, allowing for the exchange of ideas and support. This sense of community can be incredibly motivating and rewarding for both the writer and the readers.

Participation in community wellness initiatives or leading workshops is another impactful way to broaden the reach of healthy living practices. Seniors possess a wealth of life experience and knowledge that can greatly benefit their communities. By getting involved in local wellness programs, whether through volunteering, organizing events, or simply participating actively, they contribute to a culture of health and well-being. These initiatives often focus on promoting physical activity, healthy eating, mental health, and social connections, all of which are critical components of a healthy lifestyle.

Leading workshops on topics such as nutrition, exercise, mindfulness, and chronic disease management allows seniors to directly impart their wisdom and expertise to others. These workshops can be tailored to address the specific needs and interests of the community, making them highly relevant and effective. Furthermore, such involvement helps seniors stay engaged and active, providing a sense of purpose and fulfillment.

Community gardens, walking groups, wellness fairs, and health education seminars are just a few examples of initiatives that foster collective well-being. By taking an active role in these activities, seniors do not only enhance their own health but also serve as role models and leaders within their communities. This ripple effect can lead to broader societal changes, encouraging more people to adopt healthier lifestyles.

Final Insights

In this chapter, we explored how to make new habits a lasting part of daily routines. By using techniques such as habit stacking and modifying our environment, it's possible to create seamless transitions for adopting healthier behaviors. Routine check-ins and self-reflection help in assessing progress and staying motivated, while flexibility within these routines ensures that changes are sustainable despite life's inevitable challenges. These strategies make it easier to integrate new habits into our lives, promoting long-term success.

As we move forward, it's important to remember that embedding new habits requires both dedication and adaptability. Regularly reflecting on the benefits and progress can reinforce positive behaviors and keep motivation high. By setting specific goals, adjusting our routines as needed, and celebrating small victories, we can maintain a healthy lifestyle. Embracing these practices not only enhances our well-being but also sets a positive example for future generations, creating a legacy of wellness for families and communities.

11

Conclusion

As we reach the end of this journey together, let's take a moment to reflect on everything we've explored and learned. Managing diabetes is no small feat, especially for seniors who often face unique health challenges. But throughout this book, we've uncovered that it isn't about making drastic changes overnight. Instead, it's about the power of micro-habits—small, manageable actions that, when consistently practiced, can lead to significant improvements in your health and quality of life.

Think back on some of the practical tips we've discussed. Whether it's enjoying your meals more mindfully, ensuring you get up for short walks throughout the day, or incorporating more vegetables into your diet, these tiny adjustments are incredibly impactful. They've been designed to fit seamlessly into your daily routine without overwhelming you, creating sustainable habits that support better blood sugar levels and overall wellbeing.

At this point, it's crucial to focus on taking action. You've absorbed a wealth of information, but knowledge alone isn't enough. Now is the time to put what you've learned into practice. Choose just one new habit today—maybe it's drinking an extra glass of water each day, or setting aside ten minutes for a leisurely walk after lunch. Starting small not only makes change less daunting but also sets the foundation for long-term success.

You might be wondering if these small steps can honestly make a difference. The answer is a resounding yes. Each tiny habit builds momentum and confidence, gradually transforming into a lifestyle that promotes better health. By committing to just one action today, you're taking a powerful step towards managing your diabetes more effectively.

However, no journey is meant to be walked alone, and managing diabetes is no exception. Social connections and support systems play a vital role in staying motivated and accountable. Share your health goals with friends, family, or fellow community members. They can provide encouragement, celebrate your successes, and offer a shoulder to lean on during challenging times. Feeling connected to others who understand your journey will help you stay focused and inspired.

Furthermore, consider joining a local support group or an online forum where you can connect with others going through similar experiences. These groups offer a safe space to share advice, ask questions, and receive support. Engaging with a supportive community reinforces the idea that you are not alone in this journey. Instead of just surviving, let's thrive together by leveraging the strength of our collective efforts.

Looking ahead, it's important to envision the positive changes these new habits can bring to your life. Imagine yourself five years from now. Picture feeling energetic, empowered, and confident, knowing your blood sugar levels are under control. Envision yourself participating in activities you enjoy, spending quality time with loved ones, and experiencing a sense of overall wellbeing. This vision is not just a distant dream—it's fully within your reach. By sticking to your new habits and continuously striving for improvement, you can achieve the healthier future you deserve.

Remember, your health journey doesn't have a finish line. It is a continuous cycle of learning, adapting, and growing. Just as you would approach any skill, such as painting or playing an instrument, be prepared to evolve your habits as you learn more about yourself and your needs. Embrace the idea of lifelong learning, keeping an open mind to new strategies and techniques that can enhance your health.

Commit to maintaining these habits, while also exploring new ways to improve. Maybe you'll discover a new exercise routine that brings you joy, or learn about a delicious recipe that fits your dietary needs. Whatever it may be, remain dedicated to your journey of growth and self-improvement. Your commitment to continuous adaptation ensures that you'll always be moving forward, even when faced with setbacks.

Throughout every chapter of this book, our goal has been to equip you with straightforward, practical strategies tailored to your specific lifestyle and health needs. Managing diabetes doesn't have to be overwhelming or isolating. With the right tools and mindset, you can make meaningful progress toward better health. Small, consistent actions lead to big results, and the journey is far more enjoyable when shared with supportive companions.

To all caregivers and family members reading this book, thank you for your unwavering dedication and love. Your role in supporting your loved ones is invaluable, and your efforts make a significant difference in their lives. By understanding and implementing the strategies discussed here, you can provide informed support that empowers them to adopt healthier habits and manage diabetes more effectively.

For health professionals, your work is immensely important. By recommending easy-to-understand methods and emphasizing the significance of micro-habits, you can guide your patients towards improved diabetes management. Remember, the most effective approach is one that resonates with the individual's lifestyle, making it easier for them to embrace and sustain these changes.

In conclusion, I encourage each of you to reflect on the core principles we've covered. Recognize the power of small changes, take actionable steps, seek support from your community, envision a healthier future, and commit to continuous improvement. Every journey begins with a single step, and you've already taken many valuable strides by engaging with this book.

Let's move forward with determination and compassion, knowing that you have the ability to create lasting positive change. Together, we can navigate the path to better health, one micro-habit at a time. Thank you for allowing me to be part of your journey. May your days be filled with vitality, joy, and renewed hope for a brighter, healthier future.

Reference List

Adu, M. D., Malabu, U. H., Malau-Aduli, A. E. O., & Malau-Aduli, B. S. (2019). *Enablers and barriers to effective diabetes self-management: A multi-national investigation* (S. Rodda, Ed.). PLOS ONE. https://doi.org/10.1371/journal.pone.0217771

Diabetes Success Stories | UMass Diabetes Center of Excellence. (2018, February 28). UMass Chan Medical School. https://www.umassmed.edu/dcoe/diabetes-care/success-stories/

Galaviz, K. I., Narayan, K. M. V., Lobelo, F., & Weber, M. B. (2019, November 24). *Lifestyle and the Prevention of Type 2 Diabetes: A Status Report*. American Journal of Lifestyle Medicine; NCBI. https://doi.org/10.1177/1559827615619159

Hood, K. K., Hilliard, M., Piatt, G., & Ievers-Landis, C. E. (2019). *Effective strategies for encouraging behavior change in people with diabetes.* Diabetes Management (London, England). https://www.ncbi.nlm.nih.gov/pmc/articles/PMC6086609/

Laborde, S., Kauschke, D., Hosang, T. J., Javelle, F., & Mosley, E. (2020, August 19). *Performance Habits: A Framework Proposal*. Frontiers in Psychology. https://doi.org/10.3389/fpsyg.2020.01815

Michaelsen, M. M., & Esch, T. (2023, June 19). *Understanding health behavior change by motivation and reward mechanisms: a review of the literature*. Understanding Health Behavior Change by Motivation and Reward Mechanisms: A Review of the Literature. https://doi.org/10.3389/fnbeh.2023.1151918

National Institute of Diabetes and Digestive and Kidney Diseases. (2018). *Changing Your Habits for Better Health | NIDDK*. National Institute of Diabetes and Digestive and Kidney Diseases. https://www.niddk.nih.gov/health-infor

mation/diet-nutrition/changing-habits-better-health

What Are Micro Habits And Do They Work? (2022, December 13). Forbes Health. https://www.forbes.com/health/nutrition/micro-habits/

4 Tips For Reading Food Labels That Will Change the Way You Shop. (2016, February 1). Forks over Knives. https://www.forksoverknives.com/wellness/reading-food-packages-and-nutrition-labels-four-tips-for-savvy-shopping/

Cherpak, C. E. (2019, August 1). *Mindful eating: A review of how the stress-digestion-mindfulness triad may modulate and improve gastrointestinal and digestive function.* Integrative Medicine: A Clinician's Journal. https://www.ncbi.nlm.nih.gov/pmc/articles/PMC7219460/

Diabetes UK. (2017). *10 tips for healthy eating with diabetes.* Diabetes UK. https://www.diabetes.org.uk/guide-to-diabetes/enjoy-food/eating-with-diabetes/10-ways-to-eat-well-with-diabetes

Publishing, H. H. (2021, February 15). *Healthy eating for blood sugar control.* Harvard Health. https://www.health.harvard.edu/diseases-and-conditions/healthy-eating-for-blood-sugar-control

Publishing, H. H. (2012, March 20). *Cutting calories to control diabetes.* Harvard Health. https://www.health.harvard.edu/healthbeat/cutting-calories-to-control-diabetes

Reading Food Labels | ADA. (n.d.). Diabetes.org. https://diabetes.org/food-nutrition/reading-food-labels/making-sense-food-labels

Welp, B. (2023, September). *Choosing The Right Maternity Care Provider Wray Community District Hospital & Clinic.* Wrayhospital.org. https://wrayhospital.org/mindful-eating-control-diabetes-obesity/

admin. (2023, September 8). *Understanding Food Labels: What's Hiding In Your Food? - jalpashethnutrition %.* Jalpashethnutrition. https://jalpashethnutrition.com/making-sense-of-the-food-labels-whats-hiding-in-your-food/

Abushamat, L. A., McClatchey, P. M., Scalzo, R. L., & Reusch, J. E. B. (2023, January 6). *The role of exercise in diabetes.* PubMed; MDText.com, Inc. https://www.ncbi.nlm.nih.gov/books/NBK549946/

Cannata, F., Vadalà, G., Russo, F., Papalia, R., Napoli, N., & Pozzilli, P.

(2020, September 4). *Beneficial Effects of Physical Activity in Diabetic Patients.* Journal of Functional Morphology and Kinesiology. https://doi.org/10.3390/jfmk5030070

Chair Exercises For Seniors | Stone Bridge Senior Living. (2024, August). StoneBridge Senior Living. https://stonebridgeseniorliving.com/chair-exercises-for-seniors/

Felberbaum, Y., Lanir, J., & Weiss, P. L. (2023, February 17). *Designing Mobile Health Applications to Support Walking for Older Adults.* International Journal of Environmental Research and Public Health. https://doi.org/10.3390/ijerph20043611

Fabbrizio, A., Fucarino, A., Cantoia, M., De Giorgio, A., Garrido, N. D., Iuliano, E., Reis, V. M., Sausa, M., Vilaça-Alves, J., Zimatore, G., Baldari, C., & Macaluso, F. (2023, January 1). *Smart Devices for Health and Wellness Applied to Tele-Exercise: An Overview of New Trends and Technologies Such as IoT and AI.* Healthcare. https://doi.org/10.3390/healthcare11121805

Kononova, A., Li, L., Kamp, K., Bowen, M., Rikard, R., Cotten, S., & Peng, W. (2019, April 5). *The Use of Wearable Activity Trackers Among Older Adults: Focus Group Study of Tracker Perceptions, Motivators, and Barriers in the Maintenance Stage of Behavior Change.* JMIR MHealth and UHealth. https://doi.org/10.2196/mhealth.9832

Mach, J. (2024, July 14). *The Ultimate Guide to Walking Apps Tailored for Older Adults.* MedicSignal Blog. https://blog.medicsignal.com/walking-apps-for-seniors/

Wenndt, L. (2022, October 5). *12 Chair Exercises for Seniors.* GoodRx; GoodRx. https://www.goodrx.com/well-being/movement-exercise/chair-exercises-for-seniors

5 Healthy Benefits of Meditation for Seniors. (2013, September 17). Senior Lifestyle. https://www.seniorlifestyle.com/resources/blog/healthy-benefits-of-meditation-for-seniors/

Cleveland Clinic. (2022, September 5). *How To Do the 4-7-8 Breathing Exercise.* Cleveland Clinic. https://health.clevelandclinic.org/4-7-8-breathing

Dendup, T., Feng, X., Clingan, S., & Astell-Burt, T. (2018, January 5).

Environmental Risk Factors for Developing Type 2 Diabetes Mellitus: A Systematic Review. International Journal of Environmental Research and Public Health; PubMed Central. https://doi.org/10.3390/ijerph15010078

Fletcher, J. (2019, February 12). *4-7-8 breathing: How it works, benefits, and uses.* Www.medicalnewstoday.com. https://www.medicalnewstoday.com/articles/324417

Geiger, P. J., Boggero, I. A., Brake, C. A., Caldera, C. A., Combs, H. L., Peters, J. R., & Baer, R. A. (2015, September 14). *Mindfulness-Based Interventions for Older Adults: a Review of the Effects on Physical and Emotional Well-Being.* Mindfulness. https://doi.org/10.1007/s12671-015-0444-1

Kolb, H., & Martin, S. (2017, July 19). *Environmental/lifestyle Factors in the Pathogenesis and Prevention of Type 2 Diabetes.* BMC Medicine. https://doi.org/10.1186/s12916-017-0901-x

SilverSneakers. (2022). *Mindfulness meditation: The SilverSneakers guide.* Retrieved from https://www.silversneakers.com/blog/what-is-mindfulness-meditation/

Top 3 Senior Meditation Techniques. (2024). Springhills.com. https://www.springhills.com/resources/senior-meditation-techniques

A Good Night's Sleep. (2020, November 3). National Institute on Aging. https://www.nia.nih.gov/health/sleep/good-nights-sleep

Abdullrahman Darraj. (2023, November 3). *The Link Between Sleeping and Type 2 Diabetes: A Systematic Review.* Cureus; Cureus, Inc. https://doi.org/10.7759/cureus.48228

Hale, L. (2018). *Youth Screen Media Habits and Sleep.* Child and Adolescent Psychiatric Clinics of North America. https://doi.org/10.1016/j.chc.2017.11.014

Morselli, L., Leproult, R., Balbo, M., & Spiegel, K. (2010, October 1). *Role of sleep duration in the regulation of glucose metabolism and appetite.* Best Practice & Research. Clinical Endocrinology & Metabolism. https://doi.org/10.1016/j.beem.2010.07.005

Pacheco, D., & Rehman, A. (2023). *Bedroom environment: what elements are important?* Sleep Foundation. https://www.sleepfoundation.org/bedroom-environment

Sleep and Aging: Sleep Tips for Older Adults - HelpGuide.org. (2018, November

3). HelpGuide.org. https://www.helpguide.org/aging/healthy-aging/how-to-sleep-well-as-you-age

Sleep Environment: Temperature, Humidity, Light, & Noise. (2022, December 13). Sleep Doctor. https://sleepdoctor.com/sleep-environment/

8 Signs That You Are Dehydrated. (n.d.). Slidell Memorial Hospital. https://www.slidellmemorial.org/blog/8-signs-that-you-are-dehydrated

Mayo Clinic. (2022). *Diabetes management: How lifestyle, daily routine affect blood sugar.* Mayo Clinic. https://www.mayoclinic.org/diseases-conditions/diabetes/in-depth/diabetes-management/art-20047963

Nakamura, Y., Watanabe, H., Tanaka, A., Yasui, M., Nishihira, J., & Murayama, N. (2020, April 23). *Effect of Increased Daily Water Intake and Hydration on Health in Japanese Adults.* Nutrients. https://doi.org/10.3390/nu12041191

Public Health Concerns: Sugary Drinks. (2013, September 4). The Nutrition Source. https://nutritionsource.hsph.harvard.edu/healthy-drinks/beverages-public-health-concerns/

Reiland, L. (2021, July 12). *Tips for drinking more water.* Mayo Clinic Health System. https://www.mayoclinichealthsystem.org/hometown-health/speaking-of-health/tips-for-drinking-more-water

Sugary Drinks. (2013, September 4). The Nutrition Source. https://nutritionsource.hsph.harvard.edu/healthy-drinks/sugary-drinks/

Simson, R. (2021, August 9). *10 healthy ways to increase your fluid intake.* Roswell Park Comprehensive Cancer Center. https://www.roswellpark.org/cancertalk/202108/10-healthy-ways-increase-your-fluid-intake

WebMD. (2017, May 26). *What is Dehydration? What Causes It?* WebMD; WebMD. https://www.webmd.com/a-to-z-guides/dehydration-adults

Baig, A. A., Benitez, A., Quinn, M. T., & Burnet, D. L. (2016). *Family interventions to improve diabetes outcomes for adults.* Annals of the New York Academy of Sciences. https://doi.org/10.1111/nyas.12844

Chaudhuri, A. (2023, November 27). *The buddy boost: how "accountability partners" make you healthy, happy and more successful.* The Guardian. https://www.theguardian.com/lifeandstyle/2023/nov/27/the-buddy-boost-how-accountability-partners-make-you-healthy-happy-and-more-successful

Education, R. & P. (n.d.). *Accountability Partners: Don't Achieve Your Goals Alone! | Recreation & Physical Education.* Recreation.duke.edu. https://recreation.duke.edu/story/accountability-partners-dont-achieve-your-goals-alone/

Jena, B., Kalra, S., & Yeravdekar, R. (2018). *Emotional and Psychological Needs of People with Diabetes.* Indian Journal of Endocrinology and Metabolism. https://doi.org/10.4103/ijem.ijem_579_17

Johnson, P. J., O'Brien, M., Orionzi, D., Trahan, L., & Rockwood, T. (2019, January 31). *Pilot of Community-Based Diabetes Self-Management Support for Patients at an Urban Primary Care Clinic.* Diabetes Spectrum. https://doi.org/10.2337/ds18-0040

National Institutes of Health. (2018). *Social Wellness Toolkit.* National Institutes of Health (NIH). https://www.nih.gov/health-information/social-wellness-toolkit

Proctor, A. S., Barth, A., & Holt-Lunstad, J. (2023, September 26). *A healthy lifestyle is a social lifestyle: The vital link between social connection and health outcomes.* Lifestyle Medicine; Wiley. https://doi.org/10.1002/lim2.91

admin. (2023, September 14). *Benefits of Support Groups & Community for Patients with Diabetes.* Medical Market Research Blog | a Blog about Healthcare Survey. https://mdforlives.com/blog/support-groups-and-community-resources-for-patients-with-diabetes/

Adu, M. D., Malabu, U. H., Malau-Aduli, A. E. O., & Malau-Aduli, B. S. (2019). *Enablers and barriers to effective diabetes self-management: A multinational investigation* (S. Rodda, Ed.). PLOS ONE. https://doi.org/10.1371/journal.pone.0217771

Dr Good Deed. (2024, May 8). *100 Days of Healthy Habits Challenge for Transformation.* Dr Good Deeds. https://drgooddeed.com/lifestyle/100-days-of-healthy-habits-challenge-for-transformation/

Food Journaling 101. (n.d.). Cleveland Clinic. https://health.clevelandclinic.org/how-to-keep-a-food-journal

Health-Monitoring Devices and Apps for Seniors. (2024). Heritage-Rc.com. https://heritage-rc.com/resources/devices-and-apps-for-seniors

Miller, C. K. (2017, May). *Mindful Eating With Diabetes.* Diabetes Spectrum.

https://doi.org/10.2337/ds16-0039

Sugandh, F. N. U., Chandio, M., Raveena, F. N. U., Kumar, L., Karishma, F. N. U., Khuwaja, S., Memon, U. A., Bai, K., Kashif, M., Varrassi, G., Khatri, M., Kumar, S., Sugandh, F., Chandio, M., Raveena, F. N. U., Kumar, L., Karishma, F. N. U., Khuwaja, S., Memon, U. A., & Bai, K. (2023). *Advances in the management of Diabetes Mellitus: a focus on personalized medicine.* Cureus. https://doi.org/10.7759/cureus.43697

The Best Wearable Technology for Seniors with Diabetes. (2024). Seniorhelpers.com. https://www.seniorhelpers.com/mo/kansas-city-south/resources/blogs/the-best-wearable-technology-for-seniors-with-diabetes/

tfost89. (2023). *Celebrating your weight loss success without food rewards. Holistic Nutrition Therapy.* Retrieved from https://well-choices.com/celebrating-your-weight-loss-success-without-food-rewards/

American Diabetes Association. (2024). *Support for Your Health Journey | ADA.* Diabetes.org. https://diabetes.org/tools-resources

Bernardi, E., & Visioli, F. (2024, June 1). *Fostering wellbeing and healthy lifestyles through conviviality and commensality: Underappreciated benefits of the Mediterranean Diet.* Nutrition Research; Elsevier BV. https://doi.org/10.1016/j.nutres.2024.03.007

Chapter 28. Spirituality and Community Building | Section 9. Gratitude and Appreciation | Main Section | Community Tool Box. (n.d.). Ctb.ku.edu. https://ctb.ku.edu/en/table-of-contents/spirituality-and-community-building/gratitude-appreciation/main

Dr. Positive Reset Eatontown Eatontown, & Dr. Positive Reset Eatontown Eatontown. (2024, February 13). *Resilience and Renewal: How Trauma Therapy Restores Lives.* Positive Reset Eatontown Mental Health Services of Eatontown New Jersey. https://positivereseteatontown.com/celebrating-progress-recognizing-achievements-in-mental-health/

Edington, D. W., Schultz, A. B., Pitts, J. S., & Camilleri, A. (2015, September 22). *The Future of Health Promotion in the 21st Century.* American Journal of Lifestyle Medicine. https://doi.org/10.1177/1559827615605789

National Institute on Aging. (2019, May 1). *Diabetes in Older People.* National Institute on Aging. https://www.nia.nih.gov/health/diabetes/diabetes-older-people

a href='/aboutme/'>Tom Johnson. (2024, August 26). *Routines and habit stacking.* I'd Rather Be Writing Blog and API Doc Course; Tom Johnson. https://idratherbewriting.com/blog/routines-and-habit-stacking

aguilar, naudi. (2023, October 21). *The Art of Breaking Bad Habits.* Functional Patterns; Functional Patterns. https://functionalpatterns.com/blogs/articles/the-art-of-breaking-bad-habits

Also by Ranjit kumar

Thank You for Reading!

I hope you found this book helpful on your journey toward better health and wellness. If you enjoyed it and found the information valuable, I would greatly appreciate it if you could take a moment to leave a positive review.

Your feedback not only helps other readers discover this book, but it also inspires me to continue sharing helpful resources. A few kind words can make a big difference!

Thank you for your support and for being a part of this community.

Wishing you health and happiness.